A Practical Guide to Kinesiology Taping for Injury Prevention and Common Medical Conditions

Third Edition

John Gibbons

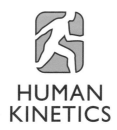

HUMAN
KINETICS

First published in 2014. This third edition published in 2024 by
Lotus Publishing
Apple Tree Cottage, Inlands Road, Nutbourne, Chichester, PO18 8RJ
Human Kinetics
1607 N. Market Street, Champaign, Illinois 61820

United States and International
Website: **US.HumanKinetics.com**
Email: info@hkusa.com
Phone: 1-800-747-4457

Canada
Website: **Canada.HumanKinetics.com**
Email: info@hkcanada.com

Drawings Emily Evans
Photographs Ian Taylor
Photographic Models Denise Thomas, Andrew Huddison
Text Design Medlar Publishing Solutions Pvt Ltd., India
Cover Design Wendy Craig
Printed and Bound Kultur Sanat Printing House, Turkey

Medical Disclaimer
The following information is intended for general information purposes only. Individuals should always consult their health care provider before administering any suggestions made in this book. Any application of the material set forth in the following pages is at the reader's discretion and is his or her sole responsibility.

British Library Cataloguing-in-Publication Data
A CIP record for this book is available from the British Library

Library of Congress Cataloging-in-Publication Data

Names: Gibbons, John, 1968- author.
Title: A practical guide to kinesiology taping for injury prevention and
medical conditions / John Gibbons.
Other titles: Kinesiology taping for injury prevention and medical conditions
Description: Third edition. | Chichester, England : Lotus Publishing ;
Champaign, Illinois : Human Kinetics, 2024. | Preceded by A practical
guide to kinesiology taping for injury prevention and common medical
conditions / John Gibbons. Second edition. 2019. | Includes bibliographical
references and index.
Identifiers: LCCN 2023015964 (print) | LCCN 2023015965 (ebook) |
ISBN 9781718227019 (paperback for Human Kinetics) | ISBN 9781913088064
(paperback for Lotus Publishing) | ISBN 9781718227026 (epub) |
ISBN 9781718227033 (pdf)
Subjects: MESH: Athletic Injuries--prevention & control | Athletic Tape |
Musculoskeletal Manipulations--methods
Classification: LCC RD97 (print) | LCC RD97 (ebook) | NLM QT 261 |
DDC 617.1/027--dc23/eng/20230518
LC record available at https://lccn.loc.gov/2023015964
LC ebook record available at https://lccn.loc.gov/2023015965

ISBN: 978-1-7182-2701-9
10 9 8 7 6 5 4 3 2 1

CONTENTS

PREFACE

I first learnt how to apply conventional athletic taping techniques while I was serving as a soldier with the British Army. At the time I was a full-time physical training instructor based at the Royal Electrical and Mechanical Engineers training establishment at Arborfield Garrison. In 1996 I enrolled on a sports therapy course with a company called Premier Training, and that is where I initially developed my passion for personal development in assessing, treating, and rehabilitating patients, especially within the sporting sector.

During the course our tutors spent a lot of time teaching us how to correctly apply tape to specific areas of the body to create the desired effect of joint and muscular stabilization. The tape we used on the course was mainly a product called zinc oxide (Z/O). This type of conventional sports tape has been designed in such a way that it has a limited amount of stretch; basically we would use this particular type of tape to help "stabilize" or even "immobilize" an area and, in particular, to correct joint positions in order to limit the range of motion (ROM). This technique aids in preventing injuries from happening in the first place, so in simple terms we were taught a method that is known as "preventative taping." We also learnt other taping techniques using elasticated adhesive

bandages (EABs). This type of bandage, as the name suggests, permitted a stretch due to its elasticity and was used to help control the amount of swelling produced after an injury. The EAB was also used to aid in compression of muscular strains and hematomas, as well as being an anchor point for the attachment of Z/O tape.

The tutors taught us many techniques during the course and, in particular, I liked a taping method known as the McConnell regimen: named after an Australian therapist called Jenny McConnell. This type of technique was typically used to reduce knee pain and, in particular, to control the alignment of the patellofemoral joint. The first taping application was to protect the skin by using a micropore tape before applying a thick piece of brown medical tape (commonly called leukotape). The leukotape was used to reposition the patellofemoral joint, and patients would typically have immediate pain relief. After the application of the tape, the patient would then be advised to do specific exercises to reactivate a weakened inner quadriceps muscle known as the vastus medialis (VM). This muscle is involved in end-phase extension of the knee joint (also known as the lock or screw-home mechanism). There are also specific fibers, known as the vastus medialis oblique (VMO) fibers, that attach to this muscle and are thought to control the position of the patellofemoral joint. This muscle and the oblique fibers atrophy very quickly when pain and swelling are present within the patellofemoral joint. If this biomechanical process happens then knee pain ensues due to a misalignment issue. However, patients who have suffered from chronic knee pain for many years would experience a reduction of symptoms and often recover simply by applying a piece of tape.

Please remember that taping techniques are an aid in relation to this area of the knee and not the total answer to the problem. When applying tape to a patient's patellofemoral joint, you are treating the "symptoms" and not the underlying cause: the application of the specific taping method will hopefully reduce the patient's presenting painful symptoms. Having initially reduced a patient's pain, you can then ascertain, through a physical therapy assessment, what might be the underlying cause and formulate a treatment plan accordingly.

The first time I actually applied tape "in the field" was shortly after finishing the sports therapy course, and I just happened to be on top of Snowdon, the highest mountain in Wales. I was leading a group of military men on a mountaineering expedition, and one of the soldiers twisted his ankle through an inversion sprain and subsequently sprained his lateral ligaments of the ankle complex: known as the anterior talofibular ligament (ATFL) and the calcaneofibular ligament (CFL). After my assessment, I decided that he had a grade 1 sprain of these ligaments and proceeded to apply a stirrup type of stabilization technique to his ankle using the Z/O tape that I had in my rucksack. The soldier managed to finish the

expedition with no further injury. Once we completed our descent from the mountain I was then able to compress the area with some ice and, when the ice was removed, I was able to use the EAB to control and assist in reducing the swelling.

In 1997 I decided to leave the British Army and was fortunate to be offered a lecturing position at Reading College to teach sports therapy and sports massage; from there, I then became a lecturer with Premier Training, the company where I initially gained my training. During my period with Premier Training I learnt a lot about all areas of sports medicine, and I gained valuable experience for which I am truly thankful.

There came a point during my career with Premier Training when I wanted more knowledge and training in other fields of physical therapy. Subsequently, I enrolled on an osteopathy degree program in Oxford and, after 5 years of focus and commitment, I qualified in 2003. During my studies to be an osteopath I decided to leave Premier Training to pursue my own dreams, and in 2002 I had the opportunity to run a sports injury clinic (Peak Sporting Performance) based at the prestigious University of Oxford's sports complex, where Roger Bannister ran the first 4-minute mile in 1954. As director of the clinic at Oxford, I have been treating the sports-related injuries of the university's sports teams, as well as the rowers who participate in the annual boat race. As a result, I have personally treated the sports-related injuries of thousands of athletes (including those at elite and Olympic levels).

For many years, and literally thousands of patients later, I was only able to use the taping techniques that I initially learnt back in 1996. However, one day I had the good fortune to meet a legend in the field of athletic taping: Ron O'Neil, an Athletic Trainer Certified (ATC) from the USA who has treated National Football League athletes. He taught me a relatively new form of athletic taping at the time known as the "PowerFlex" and "PowerTape" method and showed me some amazing techniques using this type of system. Ron explained to me that he would use these techniques to tape up an athlete before each training session and before each game as a "preventative" measure to help reduce the potential for an injury.

After being taught these superb techniques I then implemented them into my repertoire of taping skills, to complement the specific requirements of my athletic patients. My treatment now consists mainly of osteopathy, acupuncture, and soft-tissue techniques, as well as applying specific taping techniques, as and when I feel it is necessary.

I have been lecturing in the field of physical therapy and taping techniques since 1998 and have taught thousands of students to date. I particularly enjoy teaching therapists the skills required for the various athletic taping methods, as I consider the techniques I demonstrate to be a sort of an "art form"; for example, every strip of tape applied to a patient is done so for a particular reason. I always teach my students that before learning the skill of taping it is important to know the "anatomy" of the underlying tissues: in order to understand exactly which structure is being influenced with the application of each piece of tape. Once the tape has been applied it should achieve the end result it was designed to do; if not, keep reapplying the tape until satisfied and the patient/athlete is happy.

In the early 1970s, a Japanese chiropractor, Dr. Kenzo Kase, developed another type of taping system called Kinesio Taping, which was to revolutionize the field of taping. However, it was some time after his initial idea before this method became popular. Kinesiology taping was first demonstrated to me in the early part of 2000. At that time, I was not particularly impressed as it looked like a mix of colors on athletes' bodies and I personally could not see what effect it was having on the patient: it looked nothing more than a placebo effect. It took many years of experimenting with all variations of kinesiology taping methods, applied to many of my elite athletes at the sports injury clinic, before I eventually convinced myself that it actually does work. With "my hand on my heart" I can truly say, at the time I write this book, that for every single patient I have applied the kinesiology taping method to, I have never once had a negative comment about the specific application and the effect it has on them.

During the 2012 London Olympics it was visibly apparent that many athletes were having some form of kinesiology tape applied somewhere on their body. In my opinion, kinesiology taping became more obvious at London 2012 than any other Olympics, which illustrates how popular this technique has become. In addition, while researching this book, I have watched a variety of sports—e.g., rugby, tennis, soccer, athletics, and volleyball—and noted that a good proportion of the athletes use this type of taping system.

Included throughout are relevant video clips of techniques that can be accessed via QR codes the reader is able to scan the code using their smartphone and this will automatically take them to the appropriate taping technique, which is hosted on YouTube.

For those unable to access the videos via QR code, they can all be viewed on my YouTube channel, www.youtube.com/@JohnGibbons.

John Gibbons, 2023

For information on training through John Gibbons "Bodymaster Method®" certified courses on physical therapy and kinesiology taping visit the website: *www.johngibbonsbodymaster.co.uk*

John Gibbons
Bodymaster Method®

ACKNOWLEDGMENTS

I would like to thank Jon Hutchings of Lotus Publishing for again allowing me the opportunity of following my passion for writing and especially this third edition: I am truly grateful for his continual support and guidance.

Dr. Kenzo Kase, who is the founder of this phenomenal taping method: I thank you for all the time and commitment you personally put into this field of therapy. I hope that one day I have the pleasure of meeting you, as without your contribution this book would not have been possible.

To my mother, Margaret Gibbons, and my sister, Amanda Williams—I think of you both each and every day. To my father, John Gibbons (Snr)—I truly wish you were here to see my success. I miss you, dad, and think of you all the time.

Many thanks to Ian Taylor, the photographer for all my books to date. I appreciate all his extra work to make this third edition a success. Yet again he has done a fantastic job, especially with all the necessary, time-consuming editing of the photographs.

Sadly, I have to mention my son, Thomas Rhys Gibbons, who is no longer with us. RIP my little Tom-Tom … every day is a struggle for me and when I see the shining star in the sky I think of you and it keeps me going.

DEDICATION

This book is dedicated to all the students throughout the world who have attended my courses and read my books—you are my true inspiration.

LIST OF
ABBREVIATIONS

ACJ	acromioclavicular joint	**MET**	muscle energy technique
AIIS	anterior inferior iliac spine	**MTJ**	musculotendinous junction
ATFL	anterior talofibular ligament	**MTJS**	musculotendinous junction strain
BLM	biomechanical lifting mechanism	**NSAID**	non-steroidal anti-inflammatory drug
CFL	calcaneofibular ligament		
CMC	carpometacarpal	**OA**	osteoarthritis
EAB	elasticated adhesive bandage	**PFPS**	patellofemoral pain syndrome
ECRB	extensor carpi radialis brevis	**PSIS**	posterior superior iliac spine
Gmax	gluteus maximus	**QL**	quadratus lumborum
Gmed	gluteus medius		
		ROM	range of motion
IT band	iliotibial band		
ITBFS	iliotibial band friction syndrome	**SIJ**	sacroiliac joint
		STJ	subtalar joint
KTM	kinesiology taping method		
		VL	vastus lateralis
LCL	lateral collateral ligament	**VM**	vastus medialis
		VMO	vastus medialis oblique
MCL	medial collateral ligament		
MCP	metacarpophalangeal	**Z/O**	zinc oxide

GLOSSARY OF COMMONLY USED ANATOMICAL TERMS

All references to human movement are considered to begin from the internationally accepted reference point known as the anatomical position. The anatomical position is one of a person standing in an erect position with the face directed forward, the arms hanging by the side with the fingers extended and the palms of the hands facing forward; the feet are flat on the ground and slightly turned out. In the anatomical position, joints are said to be in the neutral position.

Abduction A movement away from the midline (or to return from adduction).

Acute Of recent onset (hours, days, or a couple of weeks).

Adduction A movement toward the midline (or to return from abduction).

Adhesion Fibroblast formation caused by tearing, or disruption of collagen fibers from trauma, immobilization, or as a result of surgical treatment.

Afferent Conveying a fluid or a nerve impulse toward an organ or area (as opposed to efferent).

Anatomical position The body is upright with the arms and hands turned forward.

Anterior Toward the front of the body (as opposed to posterior).

Anterior tilt Anterior tilt rocks the cephalad portion of the pelvis anteriorly with an increase in lumbar lordosis.

Aponeurosis A fibrous sheet of collagenous bundles serving as a connection between a muscle and its attachment.

Articulation A joint between two or more bones.

Caudal Directed toward the tail; inferior.

Cephalad Directed toward the head; superior.

Chronic Long-lasting (two weeks or more).

Contralateral On the opposite side.

Coronal plane A vertical plane at right angles to the sagittal plane that divides the body into anterior and posterior portions.

Cranial Relating to/or toward the skull/head.

Deep Away from the surface (as opposed to superficial).

Dermatome An area of skin supplied by a single spinal nerve.

Distal Away from the point of origin of a structure (as opposed to proximal).

Dorsal Relating to the back or posterior portion (as opposed to ventral).

Efferent Conveying a fluid or a nerve impulse away from a central organ (as opposed to afferent).

Extension A movement at a joint resulting in separation of two ventral surfaces (as opposed to flexion).

Fascia Connective tissue lying beneath the skin enveloping muscle groups and investing various organs.

Flexion A movement at a joint resulting in approximation of two ventral surfaces (as opposed to extension).

Foramen A natural opening found primarily in a bone.

Fossa A pit or depression.

Friction A back and forth movement (using digits or other) creating heat in the tissues.

Frontal plane Same as coronal plane.

Ganglion A collection of nerve cell bodies located outside the brain or spinal cord.

Greater trochanter The broad flat process at the top of the lateral femur.

Horizontal plane A transverse plane at right angles to the long axis of the body.

Inferior Below or furthest away from the head.

Insertion The site of an attachment of a muscle, tendon, or aponeurosis to bone.

Intermediate Between two structures.

Ipsilateral On the same side.

Joint The meeting of two or more bones.

Lateral Located away from the midline (opposite to medial).

Ligament A band of fibrous connective tissue joining two or more bones.

Medial Situated close to or at the midline of the body or organ (opposite to lateral).

Median Centrally located, situated in the middle of the body.

Motor Denoting axons that convey impulses from the central nervous system to muscles or glands, producing movement or secretion (as opposed to sensory).

Palmar Anterior surface of the hand.

Palpate To examine by pressing or touching.

Para- Alongside or next to.

Peri- Around or surrounding an object.

Plantar The sole of the foot.

Plexus A network of nerves or vessels.

Posterior Relating to the back or the dorsal aspect of the body (opposite to anterior).

Prevertebral In front of the vertebral column or vertebrae.

Prone Position of the body in which the ventral surface faces down (as opposed to supine).

Proximal Closer to the center of the body or to the point of attachment of a limb.

Retro- Situated behind.

Rotation Movement around a fixed axis.

Sagittal plane A vertical plane extending in an anteroposterior direction, dividing the body into right and left parts.

Sensory Axons conveying information from the periphery into the central nervous system (as opposed to motor).

Superficial On or near the surface (as opposed to deep).

Superior Above or closest to the head.

Supine Position of the body in which the ventral surface faces up (as opposed to prone).

Tendon A fibrous band of dense regular connective tissue that attaches a muscle to a bone.

Transverse plane The same as horizontal plane.

Tubercle A small rounded elevation on a bone.

Tuberosity A relatively large protuberance from the surface of a bone.

Valgus position Relates to the alignment of segments of the upper and lower limbs. Position in which the distal bone is abducted with respect to the proximal bone.

Varus position Relates to the alignment of segments of the upper and lower limbs. Position in which the distal bone is adducted with respect to the proximal bone.

Ventral Refers to anterior part of body (as opposed to dorsal).

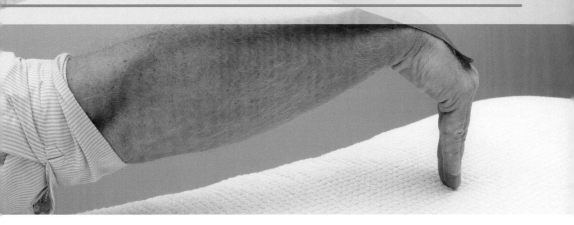

CHAPTER 1

OVERVIEW OF KINESIOLOGY TAPING

INTRODUCTION

Any physical therapist involved with assessing, treating, and rehabilitating sports-related injuries, or even patients who present with back and neck pain, will need to have the skill of taping.

Kinesiology taping is definitely the current buzzword in the field of sports medicine. This brightly colored tape is now a very common sight at all major sporting events throughout the world and is even seen at some recreational activities. Therefore, therapists need to master the techniques. They are relatively simple to learn and once applied in a specific way can improve the performance of an athlete as well as reducing any pain and swelling.

This book guides the reader toward having a better understanding of both why and when to apply kinesiology taping. It outlines how to effectively treat over 50 of the most common sports-related injuries, with the application of scientifically proven kinesiology taping methods (KTMs), and includes treatment guidelines for specific areas of the body that a patient/athlete might present with at a physical therapy clinic, e.g., lower back, sacroiliac joint (SIJ), and cervical spine (neck).

KTM techniques will be explained and illustrated for all the following areas of the body.

Plantar surface of the foot pain:
- Plantar fasciitis: proximal and distal pain
- Heel pain
- Fat pad syndrome

Ankle inversion sprain:
- Lateral ligaments
- Peroneal muscles
- Peroneal stabilization
- Self-taping

Achilles tendinopathy
- Self-taping

Calf strain/musculotendinous junction (MTJ) strain:
- Gastrocnemius
- Soleus

Medial shin pain:
- Medial tibial stress syndrome (shin splints)
- Periostitis
- Posterior compartment syndrome

Anterior shin pain:
- Anterior tibialis tendinopathy
- Anterior compartment syndrome

General knee pain:

Full knee taping for:
- Patellofemoral pain syndrome
- Patellar tendinopathy
- Osgood-Schlatter's disease
- Knee malalignment taping

Lateral knee pain:
- Iliotibial band friction syndrome
- Lateral collateral ligament (LCL) sprain
- Lateral meniscus pain

Medial knee pain:
- Medial collateral ligament (MCL) sprain
- Medial meniscus pain

Hamstring: generalized pain/fatigue

Hamstring strain:
- Medial strain: semitendinosus and semimembranosus
- Lateral strain: biceps femoris

Rectus femoris and quadriceps strain

Adductor strain

Gluteal and piriformis pain

Lower back pain:
- Lumbar spine pathology
- Facet joint syndrome
- Disc pathology
- Iliolumbar ligament sprain
- Multifidus strain

Sacroiliac joint (SIJ) dysfunction
- Big Daddy taping
- Quadratus lumborum (QL) strain

Rib/intercostal pain

Mid-thoracic pain:
- Rhomboid
- Lower trapezius

Posterior cervical pain:
- Facet joint
- Cervical muscles
- Cervical disc pain

Lateral cervical spine:
- Levator scapulae
- Upper trapezius strain

Postural taping

Pectoral strain

Shoulder pain:
- Rotator cuff tendinopathy of supraspinatus
- Subacromial bursitis
- Infraspinatus

Acromioclavicular joint (ACJ) sprain

Biceps tendinopathy: long and short head

Lateral elbow pain:
- Lateral epicondylitis (tennis elbow)

Medial elbow pain:
- Medial epicondylitis (golfer's elbow)
- Ulnar nerve

Forearm and wrist pain:
- Carpal tunnel syndrome
- Median nerve
- Tenosynovitis

Wrist pain:
- De Quervain's tendinosis
- Intersection syndrome

Osteoarthritis (OA) of the first carpometacarpal (CMC) joint

Kinesiology taping to control edema:
- Ankle edema
- Knee edema
- Quadriceps/hematoma/edema
- Forearm/compartment syndrome/ edema
- Shoulder edema

HISTORY OF KINESIOLOGY TAPING

In the 1970s a Japanese chiropractor, Dr. Kenzo Kase, started using a unique type of taping method, which led to the development of a new form of sports tape. He was keen to develop a new style of taping compared to the standard form of athletic strapping and taping, such as the zinc oxide (Z/O) technique. He felt this conventional method provided support to the muscles and joints but would sometimes restrict the range of motion (ROM), and in certain applications this technique could limit, and potentially inhibit, the natural healing process. After extensive research, Dr. Kase developed the Kinesio Taping® technique and Kinesio Tex® tape: a taping system that naturally assists in the healing of damaged tissue by encouraging lymphatic drainage and provides support to the joints and muscles without causing restriction to the ROM. This form of kinesiology taping then went on to be widely seen at the 1988 Seoul Olympics as 50,000 rolls of kinesiology tape were donated to 58 countries, which gave the taping product great exposure throughout the athletic world.

KINESIOLOGY TAPING METHOD

The KTM is another "tool" for the toolbox that can be used effectively in any sports- or non-sports-related setting. It can be applied in the comfort of a clinic or while treating an athlete at the side of the field or in the dressing room. It can even be applied to a hill walker on top of a mountain.

Kinesiology taping is not a "stand-alone" treatment as it is normally combined with other physical therapies, e.g., soft-tissue treatments such as muscle energy techniques (METs), myofascial techniques, and joint mobilizations. Once this taping system has been thoroughly understood and practically applied, then and only then, it will provide an adjunct to any treatment protocol to assist the overall well-being of patients and sporting athletes.

COMPARISON OF KINESIOLOGY TAPE VS. CONVENTIONAL ATHLETIC TAPE

Most types of athletic tape have very little or no stretch; however, kinesiology tape is very elastic and can be stretched longitudinally up to 120–180% of its original size. In addition, the thickness of kinesiology tape and its elasticity are similar to those of human skin.

When non-elastic athletic tape is applied to an injury, the rigidity of the tape can cause a restriction, or it can even prevent movement of the taped area. This is desirable for severe injuries where immobilization is necessary to prevent further damage. Most injuries, however, do not require full immobilization, and this is where the flexibility of kinesiology tape comes into its own. KTM can therefore provide support to injured muscles and joints while still allowing a safe and pain-free ROM, unlike conventional taping. This enables patients and athletes to continue training or competing while they recover from lower-back and neck pain, as well as minor to moderate sports-related injuries.

When conventional athletic tape is applied there is the possibility that circulation can be compromised, plus the issue of removing the tape after every sporting event. Kinesiology tape, on the other hand, can be worn for many days, providing support and therapeutic benefits "24/7." In addition, this tape does not cause problems to the underlying tissues or restriction to the associated joint(s). Another benefit is that once kinesiology tape is removed it does not tend to leave any glue-like residue, unlike conventional athletic strapping and taping products.

Kinesiology tape also tends to be thinner and more elastic than conventional tape, and most of the kinesiology taping products have been designed to provide "uni-directional" elasticity, i.e., stretch in length but not in width. Each company that produces a kinesiology taping product claims that the stretching capability is critical because it provides the same elasticity as human skin (even though each company claims slight variations in the amount of this perceived stretching capability: Rocktape® claims that its tape has approximately 180% stretch, and KT Tape® claims 140% stretch for its product).

Perhaps the main difference between kinesiology tape and other athletic tapes can be seen in the specific method of application (Fig. 1.1). Conventional athletic

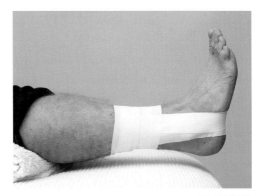

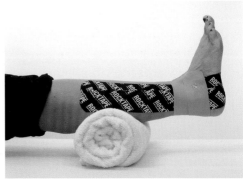

Figure 1.1 *Comparison of conventional taping vs. kinesiology taping.*

tape is typically wrapped tightly around an injured area to promote stability, and in some cases athletic tape can be applied to provide immobility. However, kinesiology tape is applied over and around the contours of the muscles and the associated joints, and the amount of stretch applied to the tape can vary depending on the purpose of the application.

TAPE ADHESION

Generally speaking, athletic tapes tend to have an adhesive applied to them that is commonly called Z/O, and this sometimes leaves a residue on the skin after removal. In addition, some patients have been known to have an adverse reaction to this type of taping system. Most kinesiology taping products that are currently available to purchase from the marketplace have a unique acrylic-based adhesive, which is normally latex-free and hypoallergenic. The acrylic adhesive is much gentler on the skin than conventional athletic tape adhesive and seldom causes skin irritation or breakdown. It does not require the use of a protective under-wrap or pre-wrap to prevent skin damage, and can be applied directly to the skin on any area of the body.

The acrylic adhesive is generally applied to the back of the kinesiology tape in a wave-like pattern that creates alternating areas of adhesive and non-adhesive so that moisture can escape easily from the taped area. In addition, the cotton fabric dries quickly so that kinesiology tape can be worn comfortably throughout showering and even swimming. A quick pat with a dry towel and it's back to its original state with no residual moisture to irritate the skin and lead to potential bacterial growth.

Even more importantly, it is felt that the alternating ridges of adhesive create a pressure differential in the tissues under the tape. In theory this will allow the tape to interact with pain receptors (nociceptors), blood vessels, and the lymphatic system to assist in relieving pain and reducing the inflammation.

TYPES OF KINESIOLOGY TAPE

There are many varieties of kinesiology taping products available on the market, and when I wrote the second edition of book in 2019, there were 70 different types of kinesiology tape.

How to Choose the Right Type of Kinesiology Tape

I have tried and tested many varieties of kinesiology tape and the top brands tested better than the easily available, cheaper options. My team and I are based at the sports injury clinic for the University of Oxford and, therefore, have been able to try most of the top brands on both elite athletes and non-athletic patients alike. All the better-quality kinesiology taping products tested well, with some variations among stretch, tape feel, adhesive quality, etc. Maybe try a few and find your own preference.

I like the phrase used by the kinesiology taping product company Rocktape (who I consider to be one of the leaders in the field). The company mentions in its literature that there are essentially two types of tape: "cheap and good tape." Rocktape highly recommends avoiding cheap tape on patients as it often peels and frays much faster than high-quality tape. Reports of skin reactions are also more frequent with cheap tape. As Rocktape suggests, I would personally avoid the cheaper and less known or tested products.

Personal Recommendations

Patients, and especially athletes, say to me on a regular basis that the main problem with wearing any type of tape—whether athletic or kinesiology tape—is the ability of the product to stay on the body during exercising. Some tapes, they complain, just fall off and refuse to stay on.

Rocktape is a company that I recommend highly and I have used its products many times on athletes and other patients (Fig. 1.2). They have various kinesiology taping products on the market and I am a huge fan of their alternative designs and funky colors, and all without compromising the effectiveness of the tape.

Rocktape also offers other versions of its standard product. There is a more waterproof form, and this is called the Rocktape H2O. This has been designed for athletes in more water-based sports, such as surfers and swimmers. They also produce a more sensitive version, called Rocktape RX, designed for the more sensitive population such as the elderly and children, because it contains less acrylic than the standard taping product. If you have larger athletes or want to cover a wider area of the body, then a 4 in (10 cm) (wide) version is available; this is also known as the Big Daddy (Fig. 1.3)!

Rocktape is currently my sponsor and the main kinesiology taping product I have used consistently over many years, both in my practice as a clinician at the University of Oxford and for training purposes on my

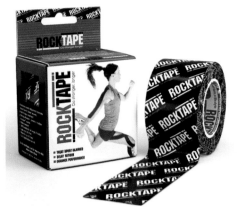

Figure 1.2 *16.4 ft. × 2 in. (5 m × 5 cm) Rocktape®.*

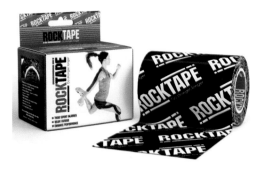

Figure 1.3 *16.4 ft × 4 in (5 m × 10 cm) (Big Daddy) Rocktape®.*

Bodymaster Method® "Kinesiology Taping for the Athlete Masterclass."

Rocktape is used for each of the demonstrations in this book, as well as the individual videos that are shown on YouTube. You can access these for FREE by using the accompanying QR codes.

Some features of Rocktape®:

- 100% cotton
- Designed in California
- Latex-free
- 170–180% stretch
- Hypoallergenic
- Water resistant
- Allows the skin to breathe

- Ultra flexible and moldable to the body's contours
- Thickness and weight of the tape are similar to those of human skin
- Easily tolerated with very few contraindications
- Allows the natural joint and muscle ROM and does not restrict motion (often a problem with conventional athletic tape)
- Elastic properties to help support and reduce muscle fatigue
- Helps assist the flow of lymphatic drainage
- Can be worn for 3–5 days without re-application
- Cost-effective patient management, i.e., 10–12 applications per roll.

HOW DOES KINESIOLOGY TAPING WORK?

Any type of injury or trauma to the body will set off the body's natural protective mechanism known as the inflammatory response (Fig. 1.4). The main identifiable signs of this response are: pain, swelling, heat, and redness, as well as restriction to the ROM.

Kinesiology taping has been clinically shown to help with the natural response to inflammation as it targets different receptors within the somatosensory system. Correct application of KTMs helps alleviate pain and encourages the facilitation of lymphatic drainage by microscopically lifting the skin. This lifting effect helps create distortions in the skin, thus increasing interstitial space and allowing a decrease in the inflammatory process for affected areas (Fig. 1.5(a, b)).

As shown with Figure 1.5a, the underlying nerve endings, lymphatic vessels, and blood vessels are in a state of "compression" due to an injury. Any type of injury will cause inflammation, as explained earlier, and this natural process will produce some form of swelling—one common type of swelling is a hematoma—and subsequently pressure will build up within the tissue. This naturally occurring process, with the increased pressure that is building up within the soft tissues, will start to irritate the nociceptors (pain receptors) and pain will be perceived. As I often quote during my kinesiology taping courses, "swelling causes pressure

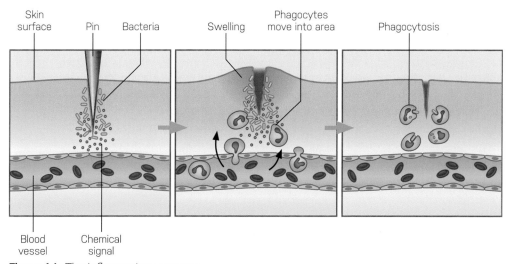

Figure 1.4 *The inflammatory process.*

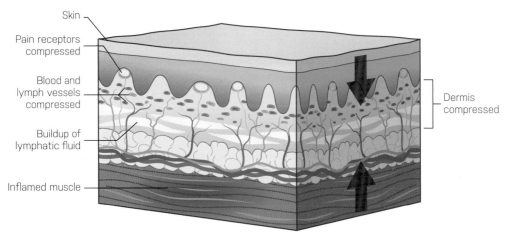

Skin
Pain receptors compressed
Blood and lymph vessels compressed
Buildup of lymphatic fluid
Inflamed muscle
Dermis compressed

Figure 1.5a *Cross-section of skin without tape applied.*

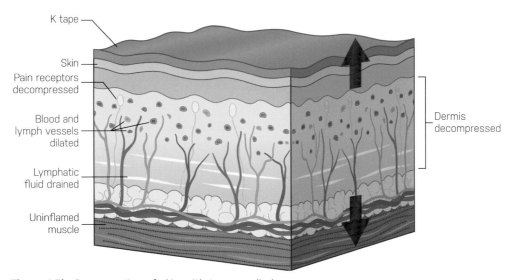

K tape
Skin
Pain receptors decompressed
Blood and lymph vessels dilated
Lymphatic fluid drained
Uninflamed muscle
Dermis decompressed

Figure 1.5b *Cross-section of skin with tape applied.*

and pressure causes pain; to reduce the pain we have to reduce the pressure, and this is where specific kinesiology taping procedures can be utilized to assist in the reduction of the pressure that has built up within the soft tissues." Other treatment methods can also be used at the same time as kinesiology taping, e.g., ice packs and non-steroidal anti-inflammatory drugs (NSAIDs).

As mentioned earlier, when kinesiology tape is applied to the skin it causes a "lifting" or "convolution" of the epidermis. This process is discussed by Capobianco and van den Dries (2009) in their book *Power Taping*, where the "lifting" of the skin is referred to as the biomechanical lifting mechanism (BLM). They state that "The BLM lifts the skin microscopically, which allows fluid to move more freely. This allows more blood to flow into the injured area, thereby accelerating recovery and repair and also allows lymph fluid to more easily drain from the area, thus decreasing inflammation."

(See Fig. 1.5b for an example of this process.)

Kinesiology taping methods have been used in the clinical setting for many years and can be specifically applied to the athlete/patient based upon their therapeutic needs. In turn, these therapeutic needs are based on the outcome of the initial physical examination and dictate the specific requirements for the kinesiology taping application, as well as other alternative treatments or modalities.

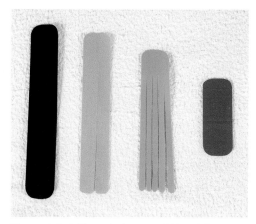

Figure 1.6 *Different shapes of kinesiology taping applications.*

HOW TO USE AND APPLY KINESIOLOGY TAPE

Kinesiology taping products tend to come in a standard size and length, normally 2 in × 6 ft 6 in (5 cm × 5 m). The therapist then decides on how and when to use this standard taping product, as they will need to pre-cut the tape for the individual patient or athlete who visits the clinic. However, some kinesiology taping products come in an already pre-cut form, which in theory makes "life" a little bit easier. My preference is to pre-cut the size and shape of the tape myself at the time of the application. This is mainly because I assess and treat a lot of elite athletes who participate in rowing as a sport, and these women and men tend to be very tall: some of the men reaching a height of 6 ft 5 in (1 m 95 cm) plus. A standard pre-cut piece of tape might be appropriate for someone who is 5 ft 3 in (1 m 60 cm) in height, but not for someone who is taller.

There are a few unique taping designs that can be created from a single piece of tape, as shown by Figure 1.6. It is very common, in all methods of kinesiology taping, to start with a single "I" strip, where the therapist will have decided on the specific length to use

depending on the height, size, and area of the athlete/patient. The standard-sized "I" strip can then be modified into a smaller version of the same strip or made into the shape of an "X" by crossing over two smaller "I" strips. The standard "I" strip can also be made into a "Y" shape or another specialized shape like a "fan." The "fan" technique is generally used to help control lymphatic drainage, as demonstrated in Chapter 9. The direction and the amount of stretch applied to the kinesiology tape can also be changed at the time of application as these will be determined by the individual needs of the athlete/patient.

Why the Different Colors and Patterns?

- Black "I" strip
- Beige "Y" strip
- Blue "fan" strip
- Pink smaller "I" strip.

All the tapes in Figure 1.6 have the same therapeutic value, regardless of color and pattern. However, depending on the sport and patient/athlete gender, the red/pink kinesiology tape is popular and is thought to be more stimulating. This color, as well as appearing to be more vibrant, is considered to stimulate certain senses within the brain and may produce a placebo effect. The blue, on the other hand, is generally considered to be a soothing color that can calm the mind and aid concentration.

How Much Stretch to Apply to the Tape?

How much stretch should be applied to the kinesiology tape? This is a commonly asked question and there are some simple rules to follow:

- **Method 1:** when applying the kinesiology tape to the patient, there is usually little to no stretch on the tape as the tissue of the patient has already been guided into a pre-stretched position prior to the application. Demonstrated in this chapter by a pre-stretch to the forearm extensors as shown in Figure 1.8.
- **Method 2:** think of this as the "decompression" strip or, in more simplistic terms, the "pain-relieving" strip. This tape can be applied with a range of 25–100% stretch, as this will help offload the specific area of pain, as demonstrated in this chapter by Figures 1.13 and 1.14.

However, there are some exceptions to the first rule of "pre-stretch" the tissue before you apply the first taping application with "little to no stretch." Some KTMs require stretching the tape as well as pre-stretching the muscle, e.g., if you want to stabilize and offload an area of pain, such as the plantar surface of the foot with a common condition such as plantar fasciitis. With this type of kinesiology taping method, as shown in the demonstration (see page 34), I place the plantar surface of the foot into a

pre-stretched position and apply between 75 and 100% stretch to the kinesiology tape. This is a typical exception to the standard first rule of kinesiology taping. This method, in my experience of kinesiology taping, works very well to help reduce the pain, even though there is no current research for this theory.

Another exception to the first kinesiology taping rule is where there is "no stretch" applied to the patient's tissue and maximum stretch is applied to the kinesiology tape. Let's take an area of the body that is very commonly injured: a sprain of the lateral ligaments of the ankle joint. The first tape should be applied at 100% stretch as the ankle has not been put into an inverted position to initiate the stretch of soft tissues. This is because the position of inversion would place the ankle in a potentially vulnerable state. Instead, apply the kinesiology tape at 100% stretch with the ankle in a dorsiflexed and slightly everted position. Then apply the tape from the medial malleolus to the lateral malleolus, as shown in Chapter 2, Figure 2.5. This technique is similar to a "stirrup" method of taping and is used to provide joint stability. To recap this technique: if applying 100% stretch to the kinesiology tape then this will assist in stabilizing the joint and, in theory, is similar to conventional athletic taping principles.

The taping techniques described in this book show the variations in the amount of stretch that can be applied to the tape, i.e., ranging from 10 to 100%. However, I personally feel that there are a multitude of ways to apply kinesiology tape and I have had the good fortune of being able to modify some of the methods I was taught. In this book I will be demonstrating the techniques that currently work for me, based on my athletes and patients.

Rocktape has another saying: "We believe there is no 'right way' to tape for any given problem." I truly believe in what Rocktape says; for an example of this you can watch, on YouTube, 15 different ways to apply kinesiology tape to the hamstrings, and you will naturally think to yourself, which technique of the 15 demonstrated is the correct one? Well, in theory, they all are correct, as the physical therapist who is applying the technique to the patient on the video is hopefully showing the technique that works for them in their clinic.

When I teach the Bodymaster Method "Kinesiology Taping for the Athlete Masterclass" I try to emphasize the following fact: it is the patient who will decide if the taping technique applied is working or not. As the physical therapist you will apply the kinesiology tape to patients in the way you were taught by your tutor. However, you will need the necessary experience and underlying knowledge of functional anatomy to have the ability to change the technique to meet the individual demands of your athlete/patient.

BENEFITS OF KINESIOLOGY TAPING

Kase et al. (1996, 2003) claimed four main benefits for the application of kinesio tape:

1. Normalization of muscular function
2. Increased vascular and lymphatic flow by eliminatination of tissue fluid or bleeding beneath the skin
3. Reduction of pain through neurological suppression
4. Correction of possible joint misalignment by relieving abnormal muscle tension and helping to influence the function of fascia and muscle.

Murray and Husk (2001) suggested a fifth mechanism:

5. Increased proprioception through increased stimulation to cutaneous mechanoreceptors.

In addition, Kase described Kinesio Taping applications for both "muscle facilitation" and "muscle inhibition" techniques. If kinesio tape is applied from the muscle origin to the insertion with stronger tension, i.e., 50–75% of its original length, this may enhance muscle contraction. However, applying kinesio tape may reduce muscle contraction from the muscle insertion to the origin with weaker tension, i.e., 15–25% of its original length (Kase et al. 2003).

KT Tape also outlines the benefits of kinesiology taping in the following product information from its website: "KT Tape is applied along muscles, ligaments, and tendons (soft tissue) to provide a lightweight, strong, external support that helps to prevent injury and speed recovery. KT Tape works differently for different injuries. KT Tape can lift and support the kneecap, holding it in place for runner's knee. KT Tape can support sagging muscles along the arch of the foot, relieving the connective tissues for plantar fasciitis. Depending on how it is applied, KT Tape supports, enables, or restricts soft tissue and its movement. By stretching and recoiling like a rubber band, KT Tape augments tissue function and distributes loads away from inflamed or damaged muscles and tendons, thereby protecting tissues from further injury. KT Tape also reduces inflammation and increases circulation which prevents muscle cramping and lactic acid buildup."

Kinesiology taping can be a valuable addition to the treatment protocol as it has been shown to have positive physiological effects on the skin, lymphatic vessels, and subsequently circulatory system, as well as having a physiological effect on the fascia, muscles, ligaments, tendons, and joints. Kinesiology taping can also be used in conjunction with a multitude of other treatments and modalities within the clinical setting and is very effective during the rehabilitative process. It can also be applied to an acute or chronic injury that has been sustained, as well as being used for preventative measures.

Kinesiology tape can be applied to the body in many ways and has the ability to assist the re-education of the neuromuscular system, reduce pain, control inflammation, enhance performance, stabilize joints, prevent injury, and promote good circulation and healing. It also assists in returning the body to its natural homeostasis.

However, it is important to conduct a physical therapy assessment of the athlete/patient as this is the key to deciding the best treatment protocol, and whether kinesiology taping is recommended. Information gained from this assessment/consultation is essential for obtaining the desired results from a kinesiology taping application, as well as any other treatment modalities.

SUMMARY OF THE USES FOR KINESIOLOGY TAPING

- Provides support for weak or injured muscles without affecting the normal ROM. This allows full participation in therapeutic exercises and/or sports training and minimizes the risk of developing compensatory imbalances or injuries.
- Activates muscles that have been weakened after injury or surgery, improving the quality of contractions and speeding up the recovery process.
- Stabilizes the area without restricting the movement like conventional athletic tape.
- The athlete and patient can remain active during the sport/activity.
- Relaxes, and can offload, overused and overstrained muscles.
- Assists the re-education of the neuromuscular system.
- Accelerates blood flow to the injured area to speed up the healing process.
- Helps to reduce pain.
- Reduces edema by removal of lymphatic fluid.
- Can enhance athletic performance and endurance.
- Corrects postural imbalance and improves the ROM.
- Inhibits muscles that are tight, fatigued, or overused and allows them to relax.
- Helps prevent injury.
- Psychological benefits as well as a placebo effect.

PRECAUTIONS/ CONTRAINDICATIONS FOR KINESIOLOGY TAPING

Kinesiology taping is generally safe for everyone, ranging from the very young to the very old and from the very fit to the not so fit. It is a therapeutic taping technique not only offering athletes and patients the support they are looking for but also enabling rehabilitation from their condition. Hence the athlete/patient can remain active throughout their sport or even their day-to-day activities.

With all types of taping methods, there are some precautions and potential contraindications you need to check before the application of the tape. Listed below are some examples (although there is no current evidence in support of this information).

Precautions

- Allergic reactions to tape
- Deep vein thrombosis and phlebitis
- Axillary and popliteal areas as these body regions are sensitive
- Local or distant sites of cancer
- Fragile skin, e.g., in the elderly or with specific medical conditions
- Skin healing in early phase.

Contraindications

- Infected areas of the skin
- Dermatological skin conditions like eczema and dermatitis
- Cellulitis
- Broken skin and wounds
- Skin reactions to kinesiology tape.

While teaching a course on kinesiology taping, I mentioned that there are very few contraindications to the use of kinesiology tape. However, there was an emergency-room nurse on the course who, while at work, witnessed a gentleman with kinesiology tape adhered to his shoulder skin, who was subsequently referred to the plastic surgery department to remove the tape. The reason behind this admission was that after his morning shower he decided to use a hair dryer on the kinesiology tape, which subsequently overheated the acrylic glue causing it to adhere directly to his skin. This gentleman should have simply patted the kinesiology tape dry with a towel. Please be careful if using an external source to dry the kinesiology tape as it is not needed and may be detrimental.

KINESIOLOGY TAPING APPLICATIONS

There are many different ways of applying kinesiology tape and the preferred style can vary among tutors. I think it is best to stick to some simple rules, and once one process has been learnt it can then be adapted according to the needs of the athlete/patient.

General rules before application

- Always check for a history of allergies to tape adhesives.
- Cleanse skin from any oil, cream, and massage wax and trim hair if needed.
- Measure and cut the tape into the size and shape required.
- Round off the corners at the end of each tape to prevent it from lifting/peeling (Fig. 1.7).

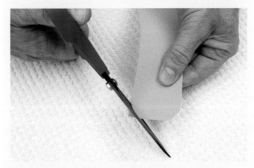

Figure 1.7 *Rounding each corner of the kinesiology tape using a pair of scissors.*

- Never stretch the ends of the tape, and leave around an inch of tape at each end that will remain un-stretched. Leaving no stretch at the ends of the kinesiology tape will avoid a "shearing" type of tension to the skin and will limit any potential for irritation, as the tape is normally kept on for at least a few days.

During application pre-stretch

Before the kinesiology tape is applied to the area that is injured, guide and place the soft tissue of your athlete/patient, e.g., the muscle, into a position that will cause the tissue to be naturally stretched, as shown with Figure 1.8 for the forearm extensors.

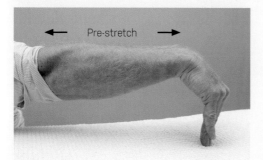

Figure 1.8 Forearm extensors in a "pre-stretch."

Please bear in mind that the patient is normally presenting with some type of pain or swelling, so only go as far as required until the patient is aware of the stretch and not to the point of discomfort.

Tape application/stabilizing technique

Before applying the kinesiology tape, expose the adhesive side of the tape so that it can be attached to the specific body area. It is natural to want to "peel off" the backing from the tape; however, this process is not needed as the tape can simply be "torn" across one of the squares as shown by Figure 1.9. This tearing will not damage the kinesiology tape as only the backing will be removed.

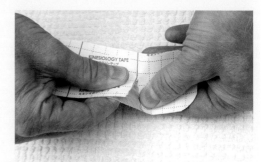

Figure 1.9 Tearing the backing from the kinesiology tape.

Apply a prepared "I" or "Y" strip to the pre-stretched tissue of the body, with little to no stretch of the tape on first application. This technique will help stabilize the area, as shown with Figures 1.10 and 1.11. There are a few variations to this rule, as described throughout this book (e.g., plantar fasciitis, ankle, and knee).

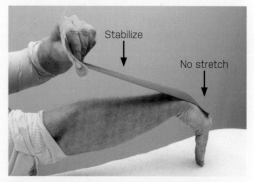

Figure 1.10 Self-application of kinesiology tape to the forearm, with little to no stretch of the tape. (The tissue of the forearm is in a pre-stretched position.)

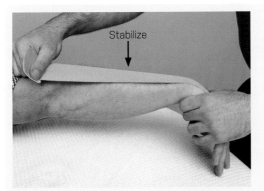

Figure 1.11 *Kinesiology tape applied by a physical therapist to the forearm, with little to no stretch of the tape.*

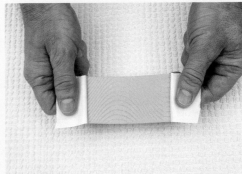

Figure 1.12 *The ends of the small "I" strip are folded back like a plaster (and no stretch is applied to the kinesiology tape).*

Pain offload application/ decompression strip

The kinesiology tape (normally an "X," "Y," or a smaller "I" strip) can be stretched between 25 and 100% of its original length. This type of application is commonly known as the *pain relieving strip* or *decompression strip* and is applied directly over the presenting area of pain.

If using a small "I" strip or a small "X" strip then it is easier to rip the backing off the tape by starting from the center of the tape, rather than starting from one end as would be the case for a longer "I" strip. Once the center has been split, peel back each end of the backing strips from the tape, and fold over the ends that have no stretch (similar to applying a plaster for a cut on the skin), as shown with Figure 1.12.

Once the ends have been folded over each other, the appropriate stretch is then applied to the center of the kinesiology tape, as shown by Figures 1.13 and 1.14.

The decompression strip of kinesiology tape, with the appropriate stretch added as

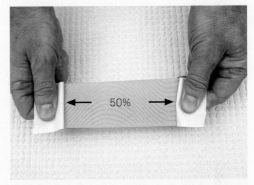

Figure 1.13 *A stretch of 50% is applied to the center of the kinesiology tape by using the thumbs.*

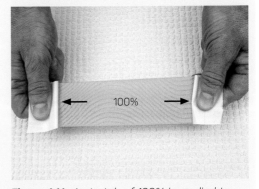

Figure 1.14 *A stretch of 100% is applied to the center of the kinesiology tape by using the thumbs.*

explained in each taping technique chapter, is then applied to the specific area of pain (as shown with Fig. 1.15).

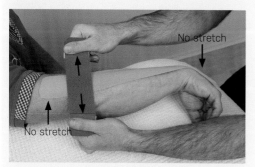

Figure 1.15 *The decompression strip is applied to the area of pain.*

Once the kinesiology tape has been applied to the area, it then needs to be heat activated (not with artificial heat) to stimulate the acrylic adhesive on the back of the tape that adheres to the skin. Do this by rubbing the tape with either your hand or a piece of the backing tape that was removed from the kinesiology tape (Fig. 1.16).

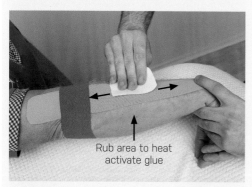

Figure 1.16 *Kinesiology tape applied by rubbing the area to generate heat and activate the glue.*

After application

- The tape will need to be removed after a certain amount of time. It is normally left on the skin for between 3 and 5 days, even though it can be removed after the specific event or activity.
- If the kinesiology tape lifts or peels at the ends then it can be trimmed.
- On removal, do not rip the tape off as this can irritate the skin.
- It is easier to remove the kinesiology tape if it is moist or even wet.
- Apply a moisturizer to the skin after removal of the tape, as this will help reduce any potential irritation.

Things to remember

- Always check for a history of allergies to tape adhesives.
- Cleanse skin from any oil, cream, and massage wax and trim hair if needed prior to kinesiology taping application.
- Stretching the structure/tissue should always be comfortable and never painful for the patient/athlete.
- No stretch at either end of the tape.
- Heat activate the kinesiology tape after application.
- Remove after 3–5 days and it is easier to remove the kinesiology tape if it is wet.
- Moisturize the skin after tape removal.

How to prepare, cut, and apply kinesiology tape

How to apply kinesiology tape

THE COLORED "STARS"

You might be wondering, especially if you have browsed through the book before reading this chapter, why there are colored stickers (or stars). For each of the individual kinesiology taping demonstrations I have placed some colored stickers (or stars) on specific areas of the body that relate directly to the pain or swelling that a patient might present with. I find this extremely beneficial, especially while lecturing to physical therapy students about the skills of kinesiology taping, as the application of a sticker enables accurate kinesiology taping.

Once the area of presenting pain has been located, then simply apply a sticker or mark the area as an exact guide as to where the kinesiology tape should be applied (Fig. 1.17). Once the area is

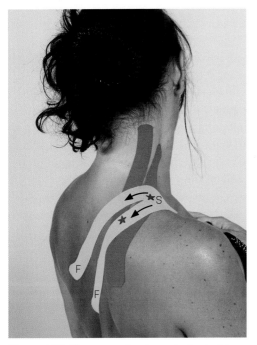

Figure 1.17 *The area of pain as indicated by the "stars."*
S = start; F = finish; and the directional arrow indicates the direction of the tape.

identified, preparation of the kinesiology tape can commence and the tape can be applied accordingly.

Reference to the individual videos using the QR code links is recommended as these explain when, where, and why I apply the colored stars as part of the kinesiology taping process.

TAPING AND FASCIAL TISSUE

A quick look through the many pathologies covered by this text will confirm the fact that most soft-tissue injuries (plantar fasciitis, tendinopathies, ligament sprains, epicondylitis, tenosynovitis, to name a few) are not to the muscle fibers themselves, but directed more to their supportive elements, i.e., fascial tissues. Thankfully, the fascia has been the focus for a lot of research over the last two decades, a fact that has given us many new insights into, and appreciation of, its many functions.

Applying tape intelligently to address fascial pathologies necessitates some further understanding of the roles performed by this tissue type. Defined as the "soft tissue component of the connective tissue system that permeates the human body," it includes all fibrous collagenous elements (Schleip et al. 2012). Its roles are to support and hold the organs and cells in place, giving them form and substance by holding them together, as well as providing both mechanical and chemical protection. The fascia provides boundaries, it contains and separates, and, perhaps most importantly for the purposes of this text, it allows movement. The fascial tissue transfers the force of muscle fiber contraction, as well as facilitating the necessary glide between structures, and is therefore especially pertinent in our investigation into injury management.

We are all familiar with the muscle epi-, peri-, and endomysia: these are the fascial containers for the muscles, the bundles, and the individual fibers respectively. These muscle fiber "bags" come together to form the tendon, which blends into and becomes the periosteum, ligament, and joint capsule (Myers 2009). These dense tissues form the major force-transmission network through the body.

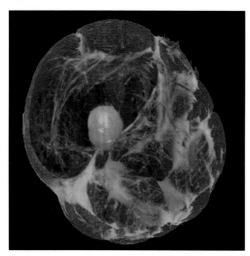

Figure 1.18 *A modern rendition of the fascial net (from Jeff Linn using the Visible Human Data Project). Here we can see the thigh. This is a small section of what could be mapped in full, i.e., the fascial webbing of the body, which would include everything from the meninges to the organ bags and supports, the muscles' epimysia, endomysia, and intermuscular septa, surrounded by the deep investing fascia and the superficial areolar and dermal layers.*

Following Wolff's and Davis's laws, the fascial tissues are adaptive and form themselves in response to the forces placed upon them. "Use it or lose it" is the general advice given for many aspects of our biology. This is particularly true of the fascia, which will reinforce itself by laying down fibers in the direction of tension and varies its makeup according to the demands of the area (i.e., stronger or weaker pulls, which may be single- or multi-directional).

The linear pull of a muscle will be the primary defining dynamic of its associated fascia, but it will also transmit force horizontally beyond its connective tissue boundary. As we can see with Figure 1.18, the collagenous tissue forms a 3-dimensional web throughout the body and is capable of transmitting force to the surrounding tissue during contraction.

This not only disperses the force but also stimulates the many mechanoreceptors situated within the fascia and forms an important channel for exchange of proprioceptive information.

A fine balance must be made between using it enough and going too far too quickly. Unexpected or unusual loads will strain the tissue bonds, leading to injury and inflammation (Myers and Frederick in Schleip et al. 2012). By applying tape in certain directions, and with the appropriate load on the stretch, we can work to reduce the strain patterns and assist with the tissue healing by protecting the area.

By applying tape, and to influence local mechanics, the therapist will also alter the strain distribution and thereby the information that reaches the mechanoreceptors (Golgi's organs, Ruffini's endings, Pacini's corpuscles, and free nerve endings) embedded within the collagenous tissues. This may increase the athlete's ability to perform certain functions if the stimulus is appropriate for them. The alteration in local proprioception should be taken into account when assessing the benefits of the application.

Between the layers of dense fascia lies a lubricating layer of areolar tissue. While this still comprises collagen fibers it contains a higher accumulation of fluid; particularly hyaluronic acid, which binds with water molecules to achieve an effect similar to silicone lubricant—imagine the necessity for the quadriceps, adductors, and hamstrings (Fig. 1.18) to all be moving simultaneously though in opposite directions or at different speeds. Maintaining the fluid content in this layer is vital for healthy movement as it allows adjacent layers to glide past each other with minimal friction. Relating the fascia to the "biomechanical lifting method" may be a particularly interesting area for future research. The lifting element of the technique may involve separating the layers to allow for a freer exchange of fluids and nutrients, facilitating the breakdown of adhesions, which can occur in these busy areas.

While taping, keep in mind the functions of the fascial tissue: force transfer also incorporates the dispersal of proprioceptive information to the mechanoreceptors and the gliding elements that allow relative movement. Understanding some of the pathology mechanisms involved in the

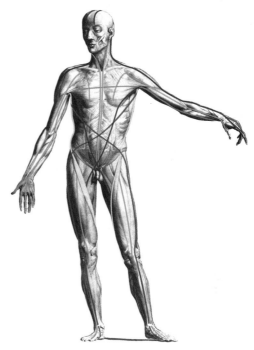

Figure 1.19 *The Anatomy Trains myofascial meridians constitute one map of how compensation can be shifted from one part of the body to another distant part.*

injury being treated may help with using the tape to create novel and individual applications. As this section can only introduce some of the ideas, further resources are given in the Bibliography.

James Earls, co-author (with Tom Myers) of *Fascial Release for Structural Balance*

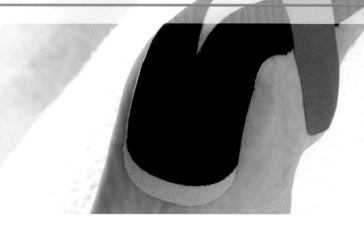

CHAPTER 2

KINESIOLOGY TAPING TECHNIQUES FOR THE LOWER LIMBS

PLANTAR FASCIITIS/HEEL PAIN/FAT PAD SYNDROME

The plantar fascia is a thick fibrous band of connective tissue that links the calcaneus (heel bone) to the metatarsals. Pain tends to present itself at the attachment to the calcaneus (Fig. 2.1) and it has been known to lead to a heel spur if left untreated. This condition is quite common and can be difficult to treat as the pain is on the plantar (underneath) surface of the foot, and the patient finds it difficult to recuperate, as they naturally have to walk.

Tsai et al. (2010) investigated the effect of short-term treatment with Kinesio Taping for plantar fasciitis. They found that if the patient had treatment with Kinesio Taping continuously for one week this provided pain relief from plantar fasciitis with a

better result compared with those treated only with physical therapy. They also concluded that the plantar fascia thickness at the insertion site might also be reduced after the application of Kinesio Taping.

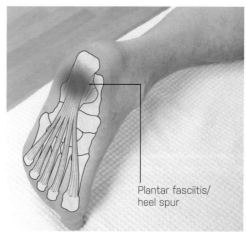

Plantar fasciitis/ heel spur

Figure 2.1 *Plantar fascia, showing the site of pain, causing plantar fasciitis.*

1. Ask the patient to adopt a prone position and place their ankle into a position of dorsiflexion with the toes extended. Anchor the "I" strip at the ball of the foot (with no stretch) and apply the tape, with 75–100% stretch, over the heel. Ease off the tape to 50% stretch as it crosses the Achilles, with no stretch at the ends of the tape (Fig. 2.2).

2. Anchor another "I" strip onto the medial side and start just above the medial malleolus (distal tibia). Increase the stretch tension of the tape to 75–100% and apply across the painful area. Ease off to 50% stretch as it crosses the lateral malleolus (distal fibula) and finish with no stretch (Fig. 2.3).

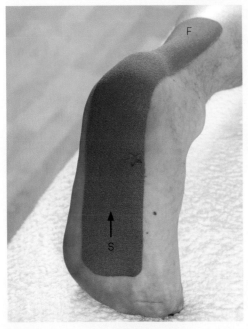

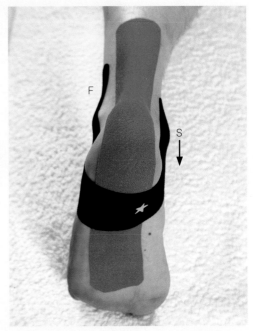

Figure 2.3 *Second taping application starting from the medial side.*

Figure 2.2 *First kinesiology taping application to the plantar surface of the foot.*

Painful foot/plantar fasciitis

3. Heat activate the glue by rubbing the area with your hand for a few seconds or, better still, use the backing from the kinesiology tape to rub the area.

ANKLE INVERSION SPRAIN/ PERONEAL MUSCLE STRAIN

Thousands of people per day twist their ankle by a motion known as an *inversion sprain*. This mechanism can stretch and even tear the lateral ligaments as well as the muscles and accounts for approximately 85% of all ankle injuries. The common ligaments to be injured are the anterior talofibular ligament (ATFL) and the calcaneofibular ligament (CFL), as shown in Figure 2.4. The muscle group that tends to be strained due to the injury mechanism is known as the peroneals.

Biccic et al. (2012) conducted a study on the effects of athletic taping and Kinesio Taping on basketball players with chronic ankle inversion sprains. The results showed that Kinesio Taping had no negative effects on a range of functional performance tests and some improvements were seen. However, the study did show that conventional athletic taping caused a significant decrease in performance for vertical jump and standing heel rise tests, while Kinesio Taping did not limit functional performance. In addition, earlier research by Murray and Husk (2001) showed that Kinesio Taping helps ankle joint proprioceptors through increased stimulation of the cutaneous mechanoreceptors.

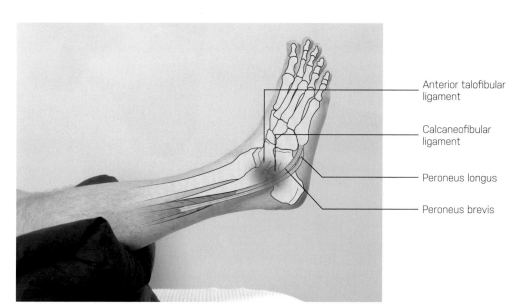

Anterior talofibular ligament

Calcaneofibular ligament

Peroneus longus

Peroneus brevis

Figure 2.4 *Lateral ligaments/peroneal muscles drawn onto an ankle.*

1. Ask the patient to adopt a long sitting position and place a towel or pillow under the calf to raise the leg. The patient then dorsiflexes their ankle and everts their foot. Once the patient is holding this position, apply an "I" strip from the medial side, just above the medial malleolus, with 100% stretch of the tape as this will promote stability. Continue under the foot and finish on the lateral side just above the lateral malleolus. Make sure that the lateral ligaments are covered, as shown with Figure 2.5.

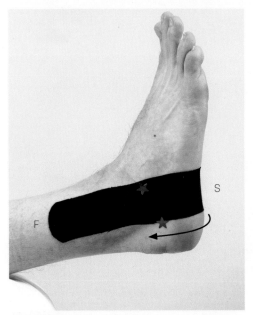

Figure 2.5 *First taping application to stabilize the lateral ligaments.*

2. Apply another "I" strip from the medial side of the calcaneus in a transverse direction, and guide the tape posteriorly to the calcaneus, so that the tape flows under the plantar surface of the foot. Apply 50% stretch to the tape and finish on the dorsal surface of the foot as shown with Figure 2.6.

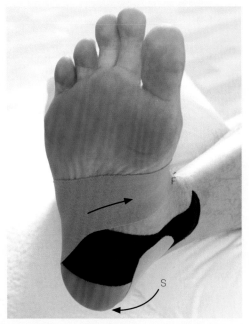

Figure 2.6 *Second taping application from the medial side.*

3. Repeat the same technique, but this time apply an "I" strip from the lateral side and, as the tape comes under the plantar surface, apply 50% stretch to the tape and finish on the dorsal surface of the foot. These two strips have a similarity to what is called a "figure 8 lock technique" as shown with Figure 2.7(a, b).

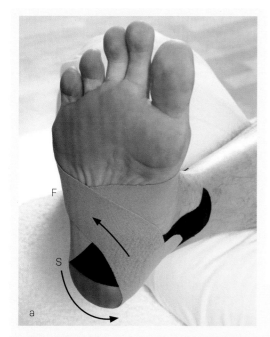

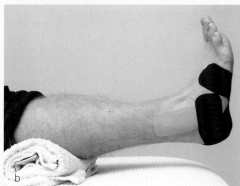

Figure 2.7a & b *Third taping application from the lateral side and finish as a type of "lock" technique.*

4. Heat activate the glue as explained previously.

Ankle inversion sprain

ANKLE INVERSION SPRAIN/ PERONEAL STABILIZATION

This technique is an alternative to the earlier one demonstrated, as the tape will still stabilize the ankle joint and ligaments; however, because I use a longer "I" strip then the peroneals will also be effectively stabilized. You can vary the tension depending on the severity of the injury; for example, week 1 you can apply 100% stretch to give maximum stability, week 2 reduce to 75%, week 3 reduce to 50%, and so on. This change of tension will hopefully allow the ankle and foot proprioceptors to start working normally.

1. Ask the patient to adopt a long sitting position and place a towel or pillow under the calf to raise the leg. The patient then dorsiflexes their ankle and everts their foot. Once the patient is holding this position, apply a longer "I" strip from the medial side, just above the medial malleolus, with 75–100% stretch of the tape, as this will promote stability of the ligaments and peroneal muscles. Continue under the foot and finish on the lateral side above the lateral malleolus. Make sure that the lateral ligaments (ATFL) are covered, as shown in Figure 2.8.

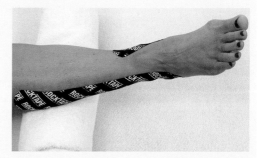

Figure 2.8 *First taping application to stabilize the lateral ligaments and peroneals.*

2. Apply another longer "I" strip from above the medial malleolus, and this time overlap the first application and apply 75–100% stretch to the tape, finishing above the lateral malleolus, making sure the peroneal muscles and lateral ligaments are covered (CFL), as shown in Figure 2.9.

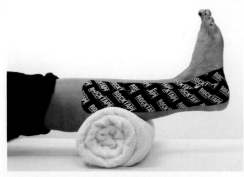

Figure 2.9 *Second taping application overlapping the first piece of tape.*

3. Apply an "I" strip in a transverse direction, starting from the medial malleolus and apply 50% stretch to the tape, finishing across the lateral malleolus and lateral ligaments, as shown in Figure 2.10.

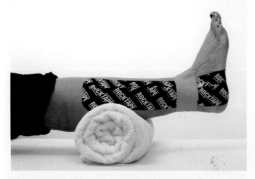

Figure 2.10 *Third taping application from the medial side, finishing across and below the lateral malleolus.*

4. The fourth application is exactly same as above; this time the tape overlaps the third application and finishes below the lateral malleolus, as shown in Figure 2.11.

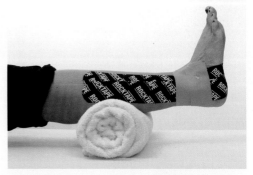

Figure 2.11 *The tape is applied in the same direction with an overlap to the third piece of tape.*

5. Heat activate the glue as explained previously.

Ankle taping and peroneals

Self-taping for an ankle sprain

I regularly teach my patients and athletes how to self-tape. Below is an example of how to apply the kinesiology tape for an ankle inversion sprain.

The patient applies the first "I" strip from the medial side of the ankle and finishes above the lateral malleolus, as shown in Figure 2.12.

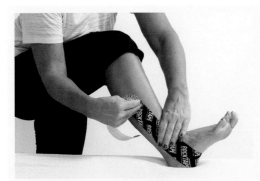

Figure 2.12 *First taping application to stabilize the lateral ligaments and peroneals.*

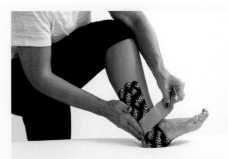

Figure 2.13 *Third and fourth taping application from the medial side and finishing across and below the lateral malleolus.*

The patient then applies a second "I" strip and overlaps the first strip, as shown in earlier figures. Next the patient applies two smaller "I" strips in a transverse direction, as shown in Figure 2.13.

Ankle inversion sprain self-taping

ACHILLES TENDINOPATHY

This is one of my favorite techniques and one of the commonest areas that I treat using kinesiology taping, as many of my athletes present to the clinic most days with some form of Achilles pain. The Achilles tendon often becomes inflamed (known as tendinitis) and mainly through overuse. It is possible to notice and palpate a thickening of the tendon over time, especially if this area is left untreated. This thickening of the tendon can change from an inflamed tendon to a potentially irreversible condition called "tendinosis" (Fig. 2.14).

Lee et al. (2012) conducted a study on the effects of kinesiology taping with athletes unable to perform sports activities due to a limited range of motion (ROM) in their ankle joints, resulting from tenderness of the Achilles tendon. They found that, overall,

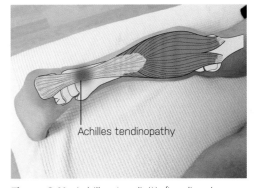

Achilles tendinopathy

Figure 2.14 *Achilles tendinitis/tendinosis.*

the active ankle ROM increased with the application of kinesiology taping. They also found, through a Victorian Institute of Sport Assessment-Achilles (VISA-A) Questionnaire*, that there was a decrease in tenderness and pain.

* Questionnaire based method that serves as an index of severity of Achilles tendinopathy.

Remember, kinesiology taping treats the "symptoms" and not the "cause" of pain. However, the technique I will demonstrate is a great adjunct to any therapy "toolbox" for reducing pain, while the underlying cause is being investigated.

1. The patient adopts a prone position and their ankle is dorsiflexed with their toes extended. Apply an "I" strip, with no stretch of the tape, starting from the heel, continue over the Achilles tendon and finish through to the center of the calf (Fig. 2.15).

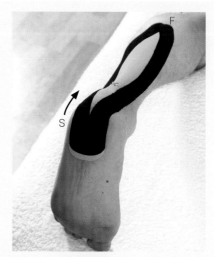

Figure 2.16 *Second taping application starting from the calcaneus.*

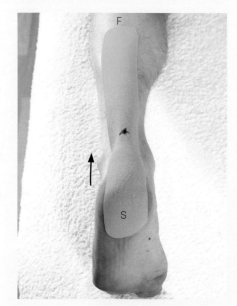

Figure 2.15 *First taping application starting from the calcaneus and finishing through to the center of the calf muscle.*

2. Apply the pad of the "Y" strip to the calcaneus bone and stretch one of the tails of the kinesiology tape to 75%. I would recommend starting on the medial side and repeating the same technique on the lateral side, as shown with Figure 2.16.
3. Apply an "X" or a smaller "I" strip across the painful site with 75–100% stretch of the tape and with no stretch at the ends (Fig. 2.17).

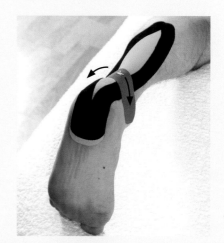

Figure 2.17 *Third taping application of an "X" or a smaller "I" strip directly across the site of pain.*

4. Heat activate the glue.

Achilles pain/ tendinitis

Self-taping for the Achilles tendon

The following technique is a self-taping technique for the Achilles tendon.

The patient is asked to place their foot on something fairly low (a couch for the demonstration) and to dorsiflex their ankle, as this will place the Achilles into a stretched position. The patient then applies the tape from underneath their calcaneus and with little to no stretch applies the tape along their Achilles tendon, as shown in Figure 2.18.

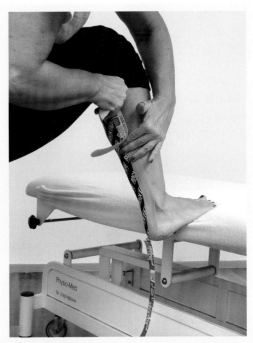

Figure 2.19 Second taping application from calcaneus overlapping the first application.

Lastly, the patient is asked to apply the small "I" strip across the painful area of the Achilles tendon, with approximately 50–75% stretch, as in Figure 2.20.

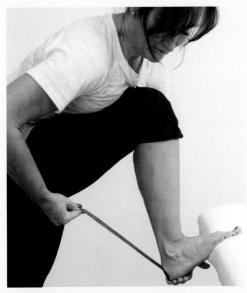

Figure 2.18 First taping application from calcaneus along the Achilles tendon.

Next the patient is asked to apply the "Y" strip along the Achilles and to overlap the first piece of tape with approximately 50–75% stretch, as in Figure 2.19.

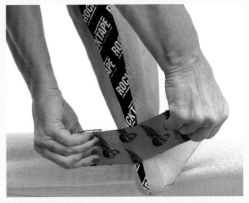

Figure 2.20 Third technique is applied with a small "I" strip across the Achilles tendon.

Achilles tendinitis self-taping

CALF STRAIN

The calf consists of a group of muscles collectively called the *triceps surae* and individually referred to as the gastrocnemius and soleus muscles. Strains of this muscle group are very common with athletes and pain is frequently associated with either the musculotendinous junction (MTJ) component, as shown with Figure 2.21, or a muscular strain/tear in the actual belly of the gastrocnemius or soleus muscle. The technique I will demonstrate works very well on both soft-tissue injuries, as the tape will help reduce the pain and inflammation.

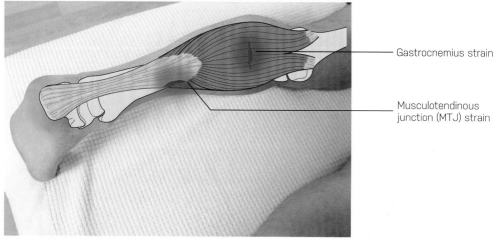

Gastrocnemius strain

Musculotendinous junction (MTJ) strain

Figure 2.21 *MTJ strain of the gastrocnemius.*

1. The patient adopts a prone position and their ankle is placed into dorsiflexion with toes extended. Apply an "I" strip, with no stretch of the tape, from the medial side, over the Achilles and across the area of pain. Finish through to the center of the calf as shown with Figure 2.22.

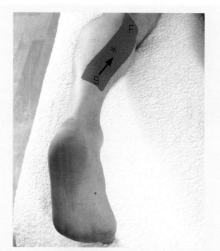

Figure 2.22 *First taping application starting from the medial side of the Achilles and finishing through to the center of the calf muscle.*

2. Apply a smaller "I" strip across the painful site with 75–100% stretch of the tape and no stretch at the ends (Figure 2.23).

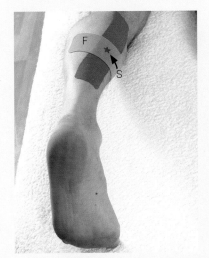

Figure 2.23 *Second taping application directly across the site of pain with a small "I" strip.*

3. Heat activate the glue.

Calf strain (gastrocnemius/ soleus)

MEDIAL TIBIAL STRESS SYNDROME/POSTERIOR COMPARTMENT SYNDROME (SHIN SPLINTS)

This is another very common condition and patients tend to present with pain that can be localized to the lower medial aspect of the tibia, especially after and during sporting activities like rugby, football, and hockey, as well as other sports. The condition starts as an irritation of the outer lining of the bone, called the "periosteum," and can lead to "periostitis." The muscles that are normally responsible for this type of pain at the medial aspect of the tibia are the tibialis posterior, flexor digitorum longus, and flexor hallucis longus (commonly known as Tom, Dick, and Harry), as shown with Figure 2.24.

If left untreated, the medial aspect of the tibia can become stressed, eventually leading

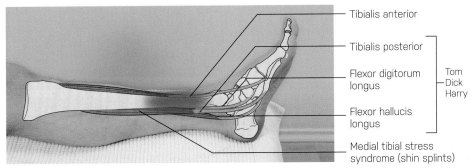

Tibialis anterior

Tibialis posterior

Flexor digitorum longus — Tom

Dick

Harry

Flexor hallucis longus

Medial tibial stress syndrome (shin splints)

Figure 2.24 *Periostitis/shin splints of the medial border of the tibia, as well as the associated muscles.*

to a stress fracture. It would take about 6–8 weeks of rest for this type of bone injury to recover before any type of training program is reinstated. In the worst case, if this injury is neglected, a posterior compartment syndrome can develop and a surgical fasciotomy to reduce the pressure within the myofascial compartment might be recommended.

1. The patient adopts a long sitting position and is instructed to dorsiflex their ankle and evert their foot to place the tibialis posterior on stretch. Apply an "I" strip from just below the medial malleolus and ideally attach the tape from the navicular bone. Apply the tape with little to no stretch. Follow the medial shin so that the area of pain is covered, as shown with Figure 2.25.

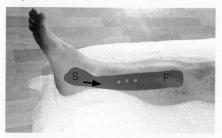

Figure 2.25 *First application of the tape starting from the navicular bone to the medial tibia.*

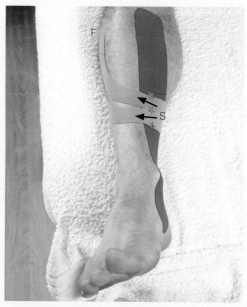

Figure 2.26 *Second application of the tape starting slightly posterior to the pain.*

2. Apply a "Y" strip, and start posterior to the pain with 75% stretch to each tail of the tape. Apply across the hotspot of the painful area, as shown with Figure 2.26.

3. Heat activate the glue.

Shin splints (medial tibial stress) syndrome

ANTERIOR TIBIALIS TENDINOPATHY/ANTERIOR COMPARTMENT SYNDROME

When athletes have pain to the anterior aspect of their shin then the following may be the cause of the problem: an anterior compartment syndrome, a strain or even a tendinopathy of the anterior tibialis or possibly one of the extensor tendons.

However, if pain is localized to the anterior part of the ankle joint then a tendinopathy of the tibialis anterior might be present; if the pain is located within the belly of the anterior tibialis muscle then an anterior compartment syndrome might be the underlying issue (see Fig. 2.27 for both of these conditions). These soft-tissue injuries tend to be relatively common in sports like hockey, football, and sometimes even running.

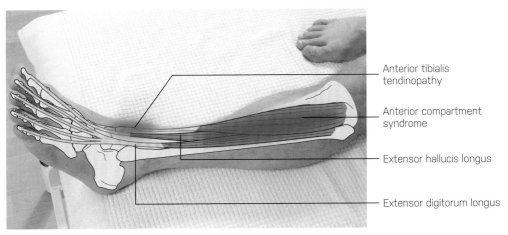

Anterior tibialis
tendinopathy

Anterior compartment
syndrome

Extensor hallucis longus

Extensor digitorum longus

Figure 2.27 *Anterior shin pain caused by tendinopathy of the tibialis anterior and anterior compartment syndrome.*

1. Ask the patient to adopt a long sitting position and to place their ankle into a plantar-flexed position. Evert their foot so that the tibialis anterior muscle is on stretch. Apply an "I" strip from the medial side of their foot onto the medial cuneiform bone and, with little to no stretch, apply the tape to follow the anatomy of the anterior tibialis muscle to its origin (Fig. 2.28).

2. Using one small "I" strip, apply 75–100% stretch to the tape and place this piece across the area of pain (Fig. 2.29).

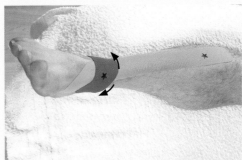

Figure 2.29 *Second application of the tape using one small "I" strip across the area of pain.*

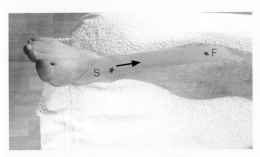

Figure 2.28 *First application of the tape starting from the medial cuneiform bone and finishing at the origin of the anterior tibialis muscle.*

3. Using another small "I" strip, place this one, with 75–100% stretch, across the area of the other "I" strip, already located across the pain, so that it looks like an "X" once completed (Fig. 2.30).

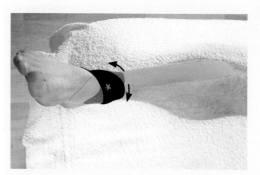

Figure 2.30 *Third application of the tape using a small "I" strip to form an "X" shape.*

4. Heat activate the glue.

Anterior shin splints

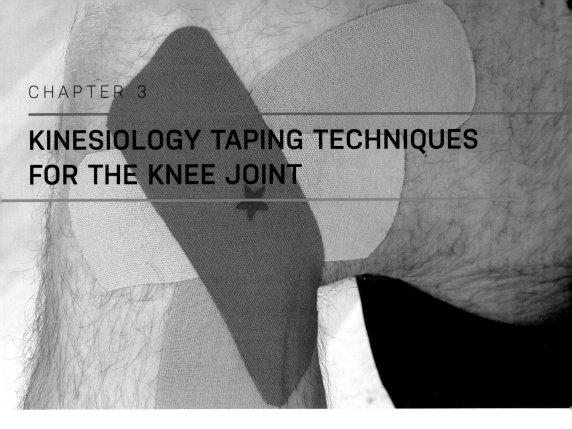

CHAPTER 3

KINESIOLOGY TAPING TECHNIQUES FOR THE KNEE JOINT

GENERAL KNEE PAIN/ PATELLOFEMORAL PAIN SYNDROME

Patellofemoral pain syndrome (PFPS) is a painful condition that can relate to a type of mal-tracking of the kneecap (patella) (see Fig. 3.1). There are many causes for this condition, such as an over-pronation of the subtalar joint (STJ) of the ankle and poor foot biomechanics. Weakness of the inner quadriceps muscle (called the vastus medialis) can also contribute to PFPS, especially the vastus medialis oblique (VMO) fibers, which are thought to atrophy due to pain and minimal swelling. In addition, weak gluteus medius (Gmed) and gluteus maximus (Gmax) can cause this type of knee pain. The knee joint is therefore what I refer to as "a weak link in the kinetic chain," and typically the presentation of the pain is not where the problem lies.

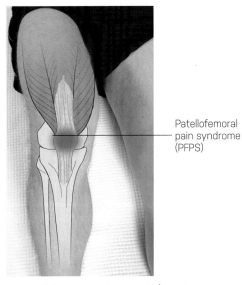

Patellofemoral pain syndrome (PFPS)

Figure 3.1 *General knee pain/PFPS.*

Chen et al. (2008) conducted a study of the "Biomechanics effects of Kinesio Taping for persons with patellofemoral pain syndrome during stair climbing." They concluded that this type of kinesiology taping could reduce pain and improve the ratio of VMO/vastus lateralis (VL) for the mechanism of patellar stability during stair climbing.

In general, PFPS is possibly one of the most common conditions that I have treated with some form of strapping and taping. This includes conventional athletic taping methods using zinc oxide (Z/O), as with the McConnell technique to control patellar alignment, as well as kinesiology taping. I like and use all the varieties of taping techniques as each of them has a unique effect upon the knee. However, my choice at the present time for helping to reduce athletes' and patients' persistent knee pains is the kinesiology taping method.

1. The patient is asked to adopt a long sitting position with their knee at 90° of flexion. Next attach a "Y" strip from the superior aspect of the patella and apply the tape, with no stretch, to the medial and lateral sides of the patella. Finish by crossing over the tibial tuberosity (Fig. 3.2).

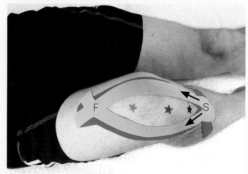

Figure 3.3 *Second application of the "Y" strip starting from the tibial tuberosity and finishing at the starting point of the first application.*

3. Heat activate the glue.
4. Once the glue has been heat activated, lower the limb back down to the couch and observe the "wrinkling" of the tape. This illustrates the effect the kinesiology tape is having on the underlying soft tissues through its unique lifting motion.

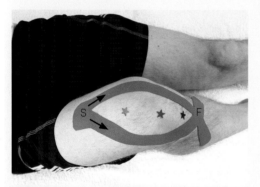

Figure 3.2 *First application of the "Y" strip starting from the superior aspect of the patella and finishing at the tibial tuberosity.*

2. Apply a "Y" strip from the tibial tuberosity and lay the tape medially and laterally around the patella so that it overlaps the first "Y" application. Apply with little to no stretch and finish near the quadriceps tendon (Fig. 3.3).

Knee pain (patellofemoral pain syndrome)

FULL KNEE TAPING: PFPS/ PATELLAR TENDINOPATHY/ OSGOOD-SCHLATTER'S DISEASE/BURSITIS

Any athlete who presents with pain inferior to the patella may also have pain in other soft tissues, such as the soft-tissue structure known as the patellar tendon. However, the pain could be due to other associated structures that sit on top of the tibial plateau, e.g., fat pad, infrapatellar bursa, and even the meniscus.

If, for example, a basketball player presents with pain to this area then it can be assumed that they have a condition called "jumper's knee," which is simply a tendinopathy of the patellar tendon. If, however, a 14-year-old footballer comes to the clinic with pain on the insertion of the patellar tendon at the attachment to the tibial tuberosity, then this is more than likely Osgood-Schlatter's disease (Fig. 3.4).

This following technique is known as "full knee taping" as it has the ability to give a

bit more stability without restricting the movement. It is an exceptional technique that can be quickly incorporated into your treatment program to offload the pain localized at the inferior aspect of the patella, as well as controlling the position of the patellofemoral joint.

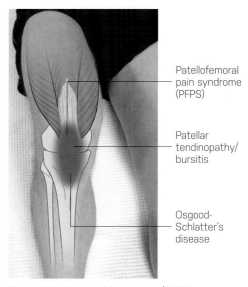

Patellofemoral pain syndrome (PFPS)

Patellar tendinopathy/ bursitis

Osgood-Schlatter's disease

Figure 3.4 *General knee pain/PFPS.*

1. Ask the patient to adopt a long sitting position and place their knee into 90° of flexion. Apply a small "I" strip across the patellar tendon at 50–75% stretch (Fig. 3.5).

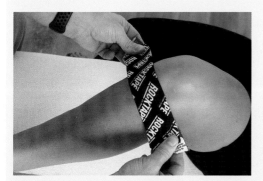

Figure 3.5 *Small "I" strip applied across the patellar tendon.*

2. Apply an "I" strip from the lateral aspect of the thigh, with a 25% stretch of the tape, toward the patella. Then apply 50% stretch from the lateral side of the patella to the anterior aspect of the knee, and finish by crossing the tibial tuberosity with no stretch at the end of the tape (Fig. 3.6).
3. This next technique is similar to the one above, but this time apply an "I" strip from the medial aspect of the thigh, with 25% stretch of the tape, toward the patella. Then apply 50% stretch from the medial side of the patella to the front of the knee, and crossing the tibial tuberosity, with no stretch at the end of the tape (Fig. 3.7).

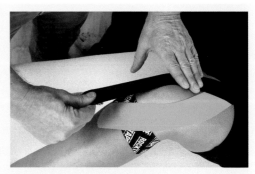

Figure 3.7 *An "I" strip is applied from the medial aspect of the thigh to the tibial tuberosity.*

4. Heat activate the glue.

 **Knee pain (patellofemoral syndrome/Osgood-Schlatter's disease)**

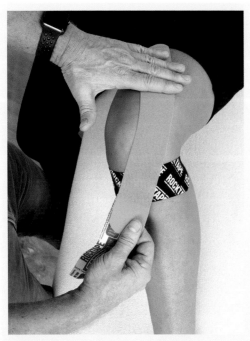

Figure 3.6 *An "I" strip is applied from the lateral aspect of the thigh to the tibial tuberosity.*

KNEE MALALIGNMENT TAPING TECHNIQUE

The two techniques demonstrated below are potentially very simple in one respect because only one piece of tape is required. I do find in practice that sometimes the simple approach can work very well. Just remember that the majority of knee pain is merely a symptom, and the causative factor for the patient's pain might be in another structure, such as the hip joint, or possibly over-pronation of the foot.

The application of a single piece of tape can be done on its own with a 2-inch small "I" strip. The technique can also be applied in combination with the full knee taping, as described below. Another option is to use the 4-inch (Big Daddy) piece of tape, as shown in Figure 3.9, in the alternative technique below.

1. Patient is long sitting with their knee straight, as this will unlock the patella from the trochlear groove and will allow the patella to be glided in a medial direction.
2. Apply a smaller "I" strip from the lateral side of the knee (LCL), and with the thumb apply a medial glide to the lateral side of the patella. At the same time increase the tension to the tape to around 50–75%, and apply over the patella to maintain the gliding motion, as shown by Figure 3.8(a&b).

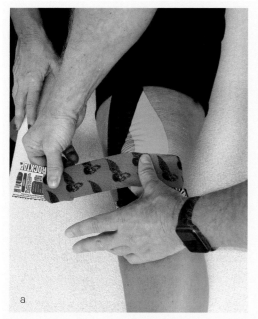 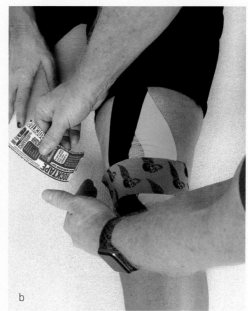

a

b

Figure 3.8 a: *Apply the tape (with tension) from the lateral side and finish medially, whilst applying pressure to the patella from the thumb.* **b:** *Finished position.*

3. Heat activate the glue.

Patellofemoral syndrome (knee pain)

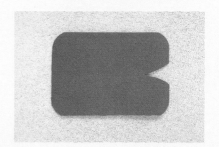

Figure 3.9 *The 4-inch tape (Big Daddy) has been specifically designed for this taping application.*

Alternative technique

This is similar to the technique demonstrated above; however, this time a larger piece of tape (4 inches—Big Daddy) is used and is cut into the shape shown in Figure 3.9.

1. The tape is first applied from the lateral aspect of the patella, near the lateral collateral ligament (LCL), as shown in Figure 3.10.

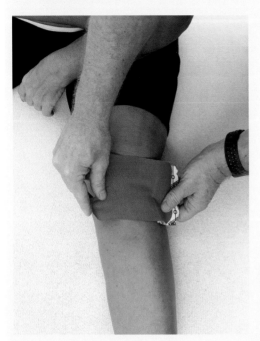

Figure 3.10 *First application of the tape, from the lateral side of the knee.*

2. With the thumb, apply a medial glide to the lateral side of the patella. At the same time increase the tension to the *superior* part of the tape to around 50–75% and apply over the patella to maintain the gliding motion, as shown in Figure 3.11.
3. Use the same procedure as above, and with the thumb apply a medial glide to the lateral side of the patella and increase the tension to the *inferior* part of the tape to around 50–75% and apply over the patella, as shown in Figure 3.12.

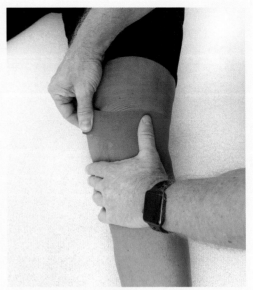

Figure 3.11 *Tension the superior part of the tape with medial glide from the thumb.*

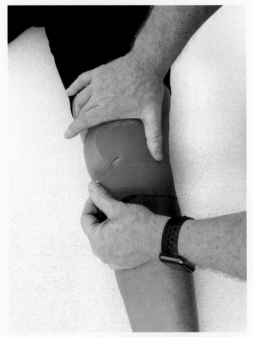

Figure 3.12 *Apply tension to the inferior part of the tape with medial glide from the thumb.*

Once you have applied the tape then the knee should look like Figure 3.13.

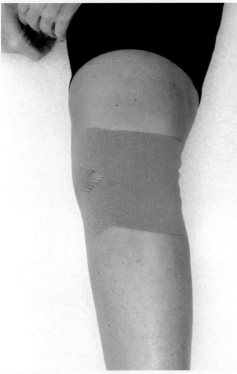

Figure 3.13 *How it should look after the tape has been applied.*

4. Heat activate the glue.

LATERAL KNEE PAIN: ILIOTIBIAL BAND FRICTION SYNDROME/ LATERAL MENISCUS/LATERAL COLLATERAL LIGAMENT (LCL)

I personally believe that everyone who enjoys running, whether competitively or recreationally, will, at some stage in their life, experience one of these conditions to the lateral side of their knee to varying degrees. There are many reasons why an athlete or patient presents with lateral knee pain and the most common reason is iliotibial band friction syndrome (ITBFS). The reason why the patient is experiencing lateral knee pain could simply be from wearing incorrect footwear, especially among those who are new to running.

It is not within the scope of this book to discuss all causes of lateral knee pain (Fig. 3.14); however, the following kinesiology taping technique will help reduce the patient's presenting pain. Through this fantastic technique, it is possible to provide enough pain relief to enable the patient/athlete to continue participating in the sport they love, as well as taking part in a physical therapy assessment (to identify the underlying cause(s)) and subsequent treatment.

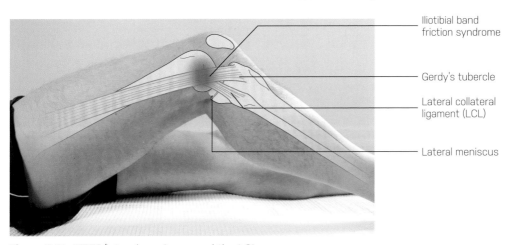

Iliotibial band friction syndrome

Gerdy's tubercle

Lateral collateral ligament (LCL)

Lateral meniscus

Figure 3.14 *ITBFS/lateral meniscus and the LCL.*

1. Ask the patient to adopt a position on their side and place their knee into flexion, while their hip is flexed and adducted so that the iliotibial (IT) band is on stretch. Apply an "I" strip, with little to no stretch, from the Gerdy's tubercle (insertion of IT band) and cross the lateral femoral condyle to finish along the length of the IT band (Fig. 3.15).

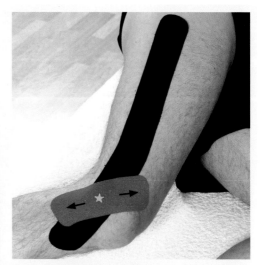

Figure 3.16 *Second application of the tape using one small "I" strip across the area of pain.*

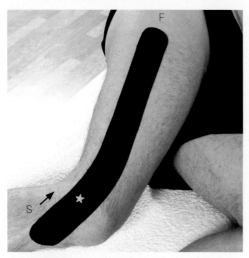

Figure 3.15 *First application starting from Gerdy's tubercle and finishing along the IT band.*

2. Using one small "I" strip, apply 75–100% stretch and place this piece of tape across the area of pain to the lateral femoral condyle (Fig. 3.16).
3. Using another small "I" strip, place this one with 75–100% stretch across the area of the other "I" strip, already positioned across the area of pain, so that it looks like an "X" once completed (Fig. 3.17).

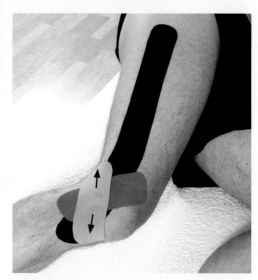

Figure 3.17 *Third application of the tape using a small "I" strip to form an "X" shape across the IT band on the lateral femoral condyle.*

4. Heat activate the glue.

Runner's knee/ iliotibial band friction syndrome

MEDIAL KNEE PAIN: MEDIAL COLLATERAL LIGAMENT/ MEDIAL MENISCUS

Medial collateral ligament (MCL) sprains and tears, as well as injuries to the medial meniscus, are considered to be some of the most common injuries, especially in sports and activities like football and skiing. The MCL, in particular, restricts the motion of a movement called "valgus." This means the knee is restricted from moving inwards, so any excessive force in this plane will often result in the ligament becoming stretched and subsequently torn (or sprained) as well as a potential tear to the medial meniscus (Fig. 3.18).

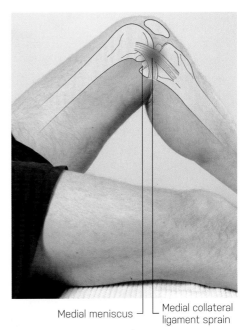

Medial meniscus ⌐ ⌐ Medial collateral ligament sprain

Figure 3.18 *MCL sprain/medial meniscus tear.*

1. The patient is asked to place their knee at 90° of flexion. Apply an "I" strip, with little to no stretch, across the medial aspect of the knee and starting from the distal inferior attachment onto the tibia. Finish on the proximal attachment to the femur, as shown by Figure 3.19.

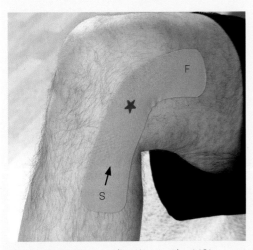

Figure 3.19 *First application to the MCL.*

2. Using one small "I" strip, apply 75–100% stretch and place this piece of tape across the area of pain, as shown in Figure 3.20.

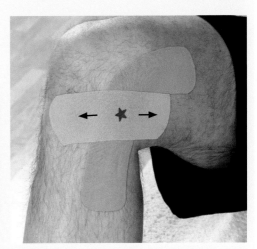

Figure 3.20 *Second application of the tape using one small "I" strip across the area of pain.*

3. Using another small "I" strip, place this one with 75–100% stretch across the area of the other "I" strip, already positioned across the area of pain, so that it looks like an "X" once completed (Fig. 3.21).

4. Heat activate the glue.

Medial knee pain (MCL sprain/medial meniscus)

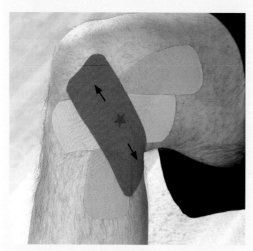

Figure 3.21 *Third application of the tape using a small "I" strip to form an "X" shape across the MCL.*

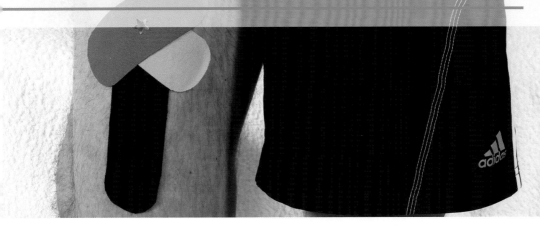

CHAPTER 4

KINESIOLOGY TAPING TECHNIQUES FOR THE ANTERIOR/POSTERIOR THIGH

HAMSTRING TIGHTNESS/FATIGUE

I treat a lot of endurance athletes, and it has been mentioned to me many times by my patients that their hamstrings (Fig. 4.1) are a constant source of pain and perceived tightness, or even fatigue, especially after a few hours of sustained exercising.

Recently I have had good success from applying kinesiology taping to the hamstrings, as this helps reduce the pain and even the feeling of tightness. I tend to combine kinesiology taping with soft-tissue massage techniques and muscle lengthening techniques, such as muscle energy techniques (METs). This system works very well for me in my clinic, especially when these techniques are used in combination.

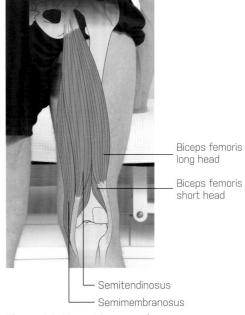

Biceps femoris long head

Biceps femoris short head

Semitendinosus

Semimembranosus

Figure 4.1 *Hamstring muscle group.*

1. Place the hamstrings on stretch and apply an "I" strip, with little to no stretch. Start from the insertion of the medial hamstring (semitendinosus and semimembranosus) at the medial side of the knee, and finish toward the origin of the muscle at the ischial tuberosity (Fig. 4.2).

aspect of the hamstring so that the kinesiology tape is applied to the biceps femoris muscle (Fig. 4.3).

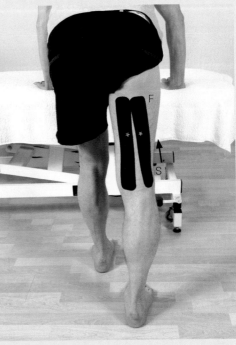

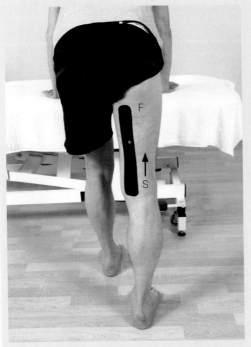

Figure 4.3 *Lateral hamstring (biceps femoris) kinesiology taping.*

3. Heat activate the glue.

Figure 4.2 *Medial hamstring (semitendinosus and semimembranosus) kinesiology taping.*

2. Repeat the same process as above but this time apply an "I" strip from the lateral side of the knee and lay down the tape, with little to no stretch, toward the ischial tuberosity covering the lateral

Hamstring muscle tightness/sciatic pain

HAMSTRING STRAIN

The next kinesiology taping technique can be applied specifically for the lateral hamstring, called the biceps femoris, or for the medial hamstrings, called the semitendinosus and semimembranosus. Through my experience I have encountered many strains of the biceps femoris and the semitendinosus. Based on this knowledge, the technique of choice is to tape the semitendinosus, as shown with Figure 4.4. If the muscular strain is on the lateral side (biceps femoris) of the posterior thigh then simply replicate the technique, but obviously apply the kinesiology tape to the lateral hamstrings.

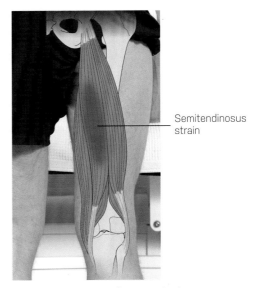

Semitendinosus strain

Figure 4.4 *Semitendinosus strain.*

1. Place the hamstring on stretch and apply an "I" strip, with little to no stretch, from the medial side of the knee. Follow the medial side of the thigh along the semitendinosus toward the ischial tuberosity, as shown with Figure 4.5.

2. Using one small "I" strip, apply 75–100% stretch and place this piece of tape across the area of pain (Fig. 4.6).

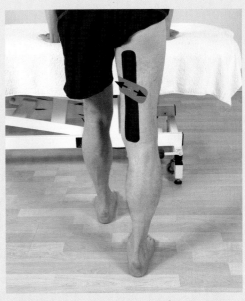

Figure 4.6 *Second application of the tape using one small "I" strip across the area of pain.*

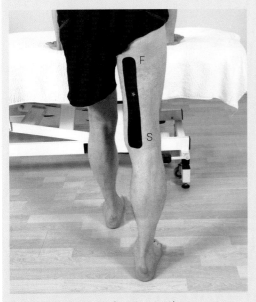

Figure 4.5 *First application to the semitendinosus (medial hamstring).*

3. Using another small "I" strip, place this one with 75–100% stretch across the area of the other "I" strip, already positioned across the pain, so that it looks like an "X" once completed (Fig. 4.7).

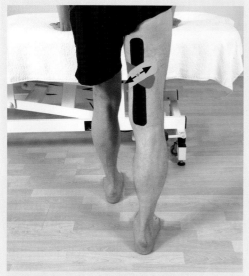

Figure 4.7 *Third application of the tape using a small "I" strip to form an "X" shape across the hamstring strain.*

4. Heat activate the glue.

Hamstring strain

RECTUS FEMORIS STRAIN

The rectus femoris muscle is often injured in sports that involve sprinting and kicking, e.g., football and rugby. However, when athletes complain of pain to the anterior thigh, it is important to rule out involvement of the femoral nerve and the lumbar spine. If muscular contractions of the rectus femoris cause pain, assume that this muscle has been strained.

Another common site of pain for patients is just below the inferior aspect of the rectus femoris origin attachment at the anterior inferior iliac spine (AIIS) and will be related to the tendon component of the soft tissue, i.e., a tendinopathy. Also, injury to the actual muscle belly or even the point where the muscle joins a tendon, i.e., the musculotendinous junction (MTJ), is regularly experienced. Figure 4.8 shows common sites of injury for the rectus femoris muscle.

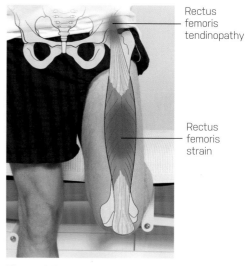

Rectus femoris tendinopathy

Rectus femoris strain

Figure 4.8 *Common sites of injury for the rectus femoris muscle.*

1. Ask the patient to flex their knee and to place their foot onto a chair/couch, so that the rectus femoris muscle is placed into a stretched position. From this position apply an "I" strip, with little to no stretch, and start attaching the kinesiology tape from the muscle insertion of the rectus femoris at the distal part of the femur (superior patella). Follow the path of the rectus femoris toward its origin at the AIIS (Fig. 4.9).

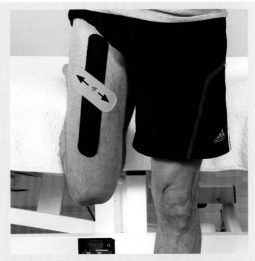

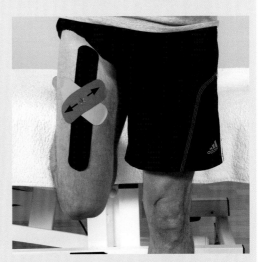

Figure 4.10 *Second application of the tape using one small "I" strip across the area of pain.*

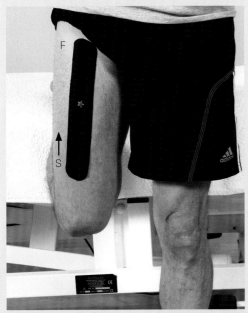

Figure 4.9 *First application from the insertion to the origin of the femoris muscle at the AIIS.*

Figure 4.11 *Third application of the tape using a small "I" strip to form an "X" shape across the rectus femoris strain.*

2. Using one small "I" strip, apply 75–100% stretch and place this piece of tape across the area of pain (Fig. 4.10).
3. Using another small "I" strip, place this one with 75–100% stretch across the area of the other "I" strip, already positioned across the pain, so that it looks like an "X" once completed (Fig. 4.11).

4. Heat activate the glue.

Rectus femoris (quadriceps) muscle strain

ADDUCTOR STRAIN

Physical therapists who treat football and rugby players in particular must see adductor strains all the time, and I personally have had my fair share of this type of muscular strain. Just bear in mind that groin pain can relate to underlying pathological changes to the hip joint, as well as a multitude of other conditions. However, if the pain is due to a muscular strain of the adductors, then kinesiology taping will help. Figure 4.12 shows a muscular strain of the adductor longus muscle.

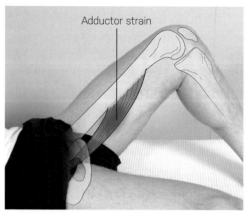

Figure 4.12 *Common site of injury for the adductor longus muscle.*

1. Place the adductors on stretch and apply an "I" strip, with little to no stretch, from the medial side of the knee toward the origin of the adductors near to the pubic tubercle (Fig. 4.13).

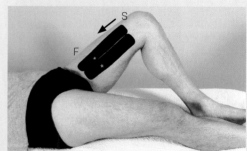

Figure 4.14 *Second application of the tape using another "I" strip across the area of pain.*

3. Heat activate the glue.

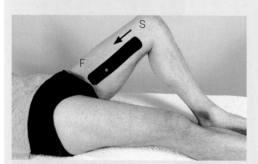

Figure 4.13 *First application to the adductor longus.*

2. Using another "I" strip, apply this to the adductors, with little to no stretch, and place this piece of tape just above and across the area of pain, similar to the first technique (Fig. 4.14).

Adductor muscle (groin strain)

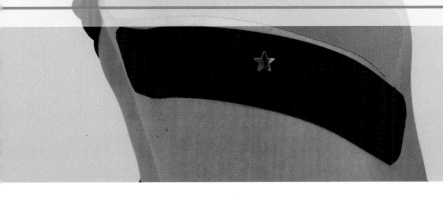

CHAPTER 5

KINESIOLOGY TAPING TECHNIQUES FOR THE LOWER BACK, TRUNK, AND PELVIS

GLUTEAL AND PIRIFORMIS PAIN

I have lost count of how many patients have presented to my clinic with pain located to the central aspect of their buttocks. Physical therapists will have their own hypotheses on what is causing the patient's presenting pain: perhaps the pain is coming from an area of the lumbar spine, such as a facet joint, or perhaps it could even be coming from a lumbar spine disc pathology that is contacting one of the exiting nerve roots. I have even seen a posterior "labral" tear of the hip joint that caused buttock pain, so please be aware that it might not be simply the "piriformis" muscle that is causing the patient's presenting pain. Just keep this in mind the next time a patient presents with pain located in their buttocks and says they have been told they have piriformis syndrome.

Figure 5.1 shows areas of the buttocks that could be responsible for the presenting pain: the piriformis, gluteals, sciatic nerve, or even referred pain from the lumbar spine, just to name a few.

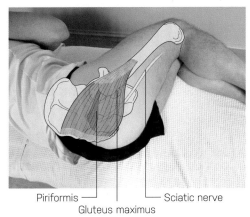

Piriformis — ┃ ┃ ┗— Sciatic nerve
Gluteus maximus

Figure 5.1 *Common causes for pain within the buttocks.*

1. Place the piriformis on stretch by asking the patient to lie on their side and bring their hip and knee into flexion. Expose this area of the body and apply an "I" strip, with up to 25% stretch. Start from the origin of the piriformis at the sacrum and apply the "I" strip toward the greater trochanter, as shown by Figure 5.2.

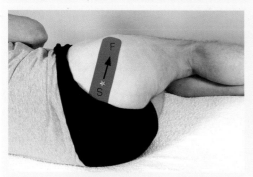

Figure 5.2 *First application to the piriformis.*

2. Apply one small "I" strip across the area of pain with 75–100% stretch (Fig. 5.3).

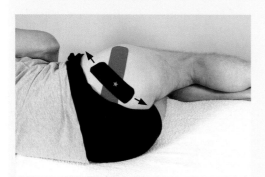

Figure 5.3 *Second application of the tape across the area of pain with one "I" strip.*

3. Apply another small "I" strip across the area of pain with 75–100% stretch (Fig. 5.4).

Figure 5.4 *Third application of the tape across the area of pain with one "I" strip so that an "X" shape is formed.*

4. Heat activate the glue.

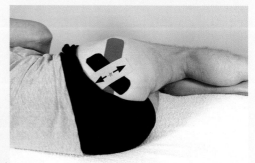

Piriformis syndrome/ gluteal pain

LUMBAR SPINE PATHOLOGY

Many of the athletes and patients who visit my clinic have pain located to the lower back, sacroiliac joint (SIJ), or neck (cervical area). Therefore, the lower back is one of the commonest areas that I treat, and, as four out of five patients will have back pain at some point in their lives, it is a good idea for physical therapists to become familiar with assessing and treating this region. Kinesiology taping, in my experience, works very well for stabilizing this area, as well as helping to reduce patients' pain. Figure 5.5 shows some common sites of pain localized to the lower back.

Yoshida and Kahanov (2007) performed a study to determine the effects of Kinesio Taping on ranges of motion (ROMs) of the trunk. They concluded that the Kinesio Taping group achieved a gain of 7 in (17.8 cm) for trunk flexion compared to the non–Kinesio Taping group. However, side bending and extension showed no improvement in the ROM with the application of Kinesio Taping.

In addition, Castro-Sanchez et al. (2012) studied the effect of Kinesio Taping in reducing disability and pain in chronic nonspecific low-back pain. They found that individuals experienced significant improvements immediately after the application of Kinesio Taping, in the following categories: disability, pain, isometric endurance of the trunk muscles, and perhaps even trunk flexion ROM.

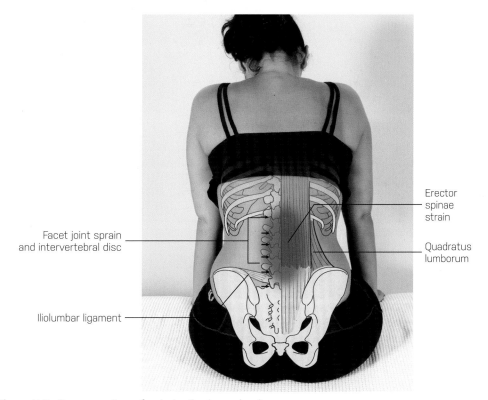

Erector spinae strain

Quadratus lumborum

Facet joint sprain and intervertebral disc

Iliolumbar ligament

Figure 5.5 *Common sites of pain to the lower back.*

1. Place the trunk into flexion. Apply two standard "I" strips across the lower back with 75% stretch to each strip (Fig. 5.6).

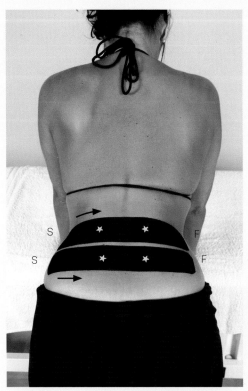

Figure 5.6 *First application of two "I" strips across the lower back.*

2. Apply two standard "I" strips, one at a time, starting from the posterior superior iliac spine (PSIS) area of the ilium. Apply up the lumbar spine erector spinae (cephalad) with 75% stretch to each strip (Fig. 5.7).

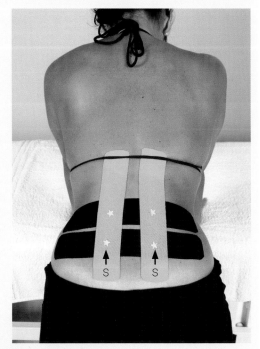

Figure 5.7 *Second application of two "I" strips up the erector spinae.*

3. Heat activate the glue.

Lower back pain/ sacroiliac joint

SACROILIAC JOINT DYSFUNCTION

Pain that is isolated to the inferior lateral aspect of the lower back might be coming from the SIJ. This is a very common area of pain with all types of patients, not just those who are active.

The SIJ, as shown by Figure 5.8, can be helped by the following kinesiology taping technique, especially if the pain is very acute and the patient is in too much discomfort for traditional types of treatment: mobilizations and soft-tissue massage.

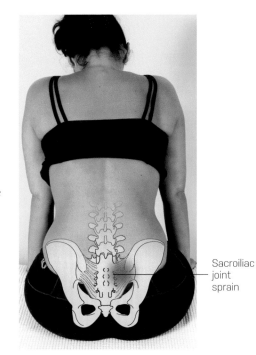

Sacroiliac joint sprain

Figure 5.8 *SIJ dysfunction.*

1. Place the trunk into flexion and rotation to the opposite side to the pain, so that the SIJ is placed under stretch. Start from the inferior aspect of the PSIS and apply a standard "I" strip in a cephalad direction, so that it crosses the sacroiliac joint with 75% stretch (Fig. 5.9).
2. Apply another standard "I" strip in a transverse direction and with 75% stretch (Fig. 5.10).
3. Apply a third standard "I" strip on the diagonal with 75% stretch (Fig. 5.11). A further "I" strip may be applied on the opposite diagonal, if desired, to form a "star" shape.
4. Heat activate the glue.

Sacroiliac joint and lower back pain

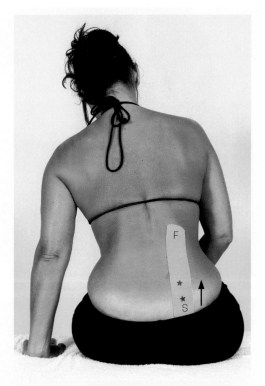

Figure 5.9 *First application of an "I" strip applied in a cephalad direction across the SIJ.*

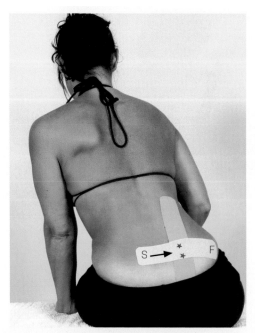

Figure 5.10 *Second application of another "I" strip across the SIJ.*

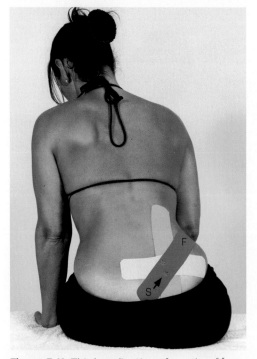

Figure 5.11 *Third application of another "I" strip across the SIJ.*

The lumbar spine and SIJ have already been mentioned; however, another choice of taping will be through the use of the 4-inch (Big Daddy) tape, as this will cover a larger area of the body and will naturally reduce the overall time taken to apply the tape, because only one piece of tape is used.

1. Place the trunk into flexion. Split the center of the tape and apply the tape to the central part of the lumbar spine. Next peel back one side, tension the tape to approximately 50–75% stretch, and then lay it down across the lower back as shown in Figure 5.12.

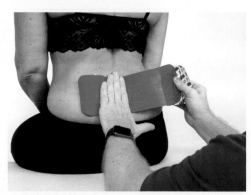

Figure 5.12 *Big Daddy tape applied to one side of the body with 50–75% stretch.*

2. Peel back the other side, tension the tape to approximately 50–75% stretch, and then lay it down across the other side of the lower back, as shown in Figure 5.13 (a&b).
3. Heat activate the glue.

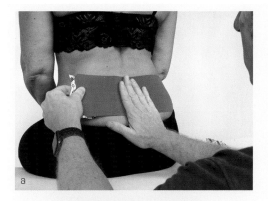

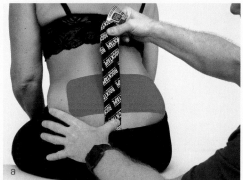

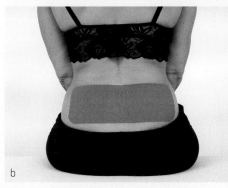

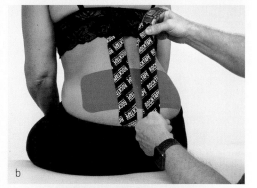

Figure 5.13 a: *Big Daddy tape applied to the other side of the body with 50–75% stretch.* **b:** *Finished technique.*

Alternative option

As a choice you can simply leave the Big Daddy tape on as it is; however, what I find in my practice is that certain patients feel like they need a little more stability. If that is the case then the following technique is recommended.

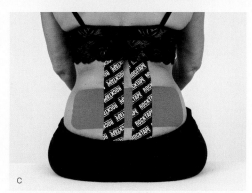

Figure 5.14 a: *The left side having the tape applied.* **b:** *The right side.* **c:** *The finished technique.*

1. Apply two standard "I" strips, one at a time, starting from the posterior superior iliac spine (PSIS) area of the ilium. Apply up the lumbar spine erector spinae (cephalad) with 50–75% stretch to each strip, as shown in Figure 5.14 (a,b,&c).
2. Heat activate the glue.

Lumbar spine pain (using Big Daddy)

QUADRATUS LUMBORUM (QL) STRAIN

Earlier (Fig. 5.5) the quadratus lumborum (QL) was mentioned, so it would make sense to have a specific taping technique for this unique muscle.

1. Place the trunk into lateral flexion. Apply two standard "I" strips, one at a time, starting from the iliac crest and apply laterally toward the lumbar spine and across the QL muscle with 50–75% stretch to each strip, as shown in Figure 5.15 (a&b).

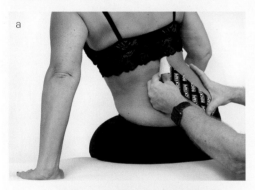

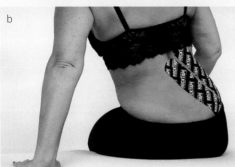

Figure 5.15 a: *First "I" strip applied laterally across the QL muscle with 50–75% stretch.* **b:** *Second "I" strip applied.*

2. Next apply two standard "I" strips, one at a time, the first starting from the PSIS and the second from the lumbar spine, and apply laterally across the QL

muscle toward the lower ribs and with 50–75% stretch to each strip, as shown in Figure 5.15 (c&d).

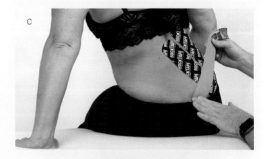

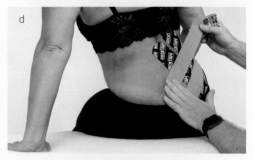

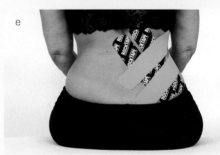

Figure 5.15 c: *First "I" strip applied from the PSIS laterally across the QL muscle with 50–75% stretch.* **d:** *Second "I" strip applied from lumbar spine to lower ribs.* **e:** *Finished application.*

3. Heat activate the glue.

Lower back pain/ quadratus lumborum

RIB/INTERCOSTAL PAIN

Rib stress fractures are a rare occurrence unless training at least 12–14 sessions per week, like the elite rowing teams, or sustained from a direct blow, as may occur in contact sports such as football. As a physical therapist I have seen many rib stress fractures in my time at Oxford, especially as I have been treating Olympic and elite-level rowers for many years. At the end of the day, if a bone scan confirms the diagnosis of a stress fracture, nature is by far the best healer (Fig. 5.16). It will generally take around six weeks, at least, to heal, and hopefully the application of the kinesiology tape might speed up this process. However, there is no current research to confirm this. If the pain is located to the intercostal muscles, then the following taping application can reduce discomfort immensely.

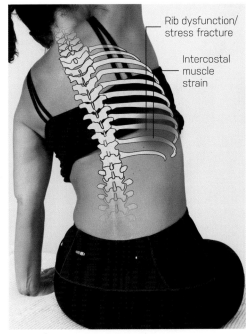

Rib dysfunction/ stress fracture

Intercostal muscle strain

Figure 5.16 *Common sites of pain localized to the area of the ribs.*

1. Place the trunk into side bending with the arm raised above the head to the opposite side from the pain, so that the ribs are placed under stretch. Apply a standard "I" strip superior to the area of pain and follow the alignment of the rib with 10–15% stretch of the tape (Fig. 5.17).
2. Apply another standard "I" strip in a transverse direction inferior to the area of pain and with 10–15% stretch (Fig. 5.18).

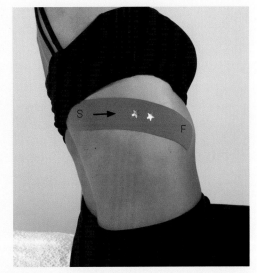

Figure 5.17 *First application of an "I" strip superior to the area of the rib pain.*

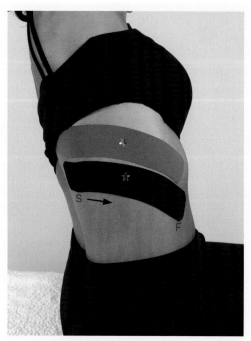

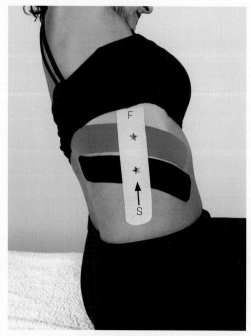

Figure 5.18 *Second application of an "I" strip inferior to the area of the rib pain.*

Figure 5.19 *Third application of an "I" strip crossing the area of rib pain.*

3. Apply a third standard "I" strip, with 10–15% stretch, starting from above the iliac crest and toward the axilla, so that the area of pain is crossed (Fig. 5.19).

4. Heat activate the glue.

Intercostal muscles and rib pain

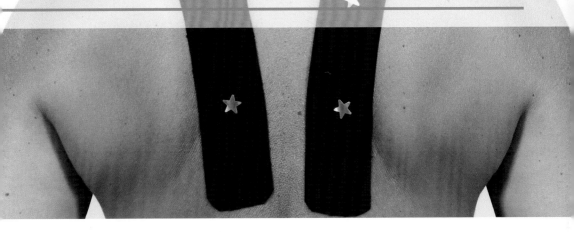

CHAPTER 6

KINESIOLOGY TAPING FOR THE UPPER BACK, NECK, AND CHEST

MID-THORACIC AND RHOMBOID PAIN

Karatas et al. (2012) found, through their study of surgeons who presented with musculoskeletal pain, that Kinesio Taping made a significant improvement to the range of motion (ROM) of the cervical spine as well as providing a reduction in pain. They concluded that Kinesio Taping would be an effective method for reducing neck and lower back pain and improving cervical and lumbar ROM and functional performance.

Pain that presents itself to the mid-thoracic region between the shoulder blades (scapulae) is possibly due to either a strain of the rhomboid or the lower trapezius muscle (Fig. 6.1). The pain may also be referred and potentially coming from the lower cervical spine. It is also essential to consider a rib or a thoracic spine dysfunction as part of the differential diagnosis. Rarely, the symptoms might also suggest an issue from the lungs or the intercostal muscles.

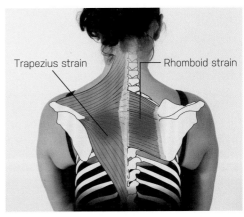

Figure 6.1 *Mid-thoracic muscles (rhomboids and trapezius).*

Many patients who come to the clinic have postural issues so that the mid-thoracic muscles are continually on stretch; this could be due to shortened and tight antagonistic (opposite) muscles of the pectoralis major and minor. Treatment should include some muscle lengthening techniques of the pectorals rather than just treating where it hurts: as "where the pain is the problem is not," to quote from Dr. Ida Rolf, founder of the technique Rolfing.

Kinesiology taping for this type of condition is an excellent adjunct to the treatment program as it makes the patient aware of their posture and inclined to do the recommended exercises.

1. Place the mid-trunk into flexion and ask the patient to protract their shoulders so that the mid-thoracic muscles are on stretch. Apply two standard "I" strips, one at a time, starting from the upper trapezius. Continue caudally along the erector spinae muscles with 75% stretch to each strip (Fig. 6.2).

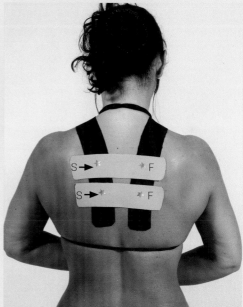

Figure 6.3 *Second application of two "I" strips between the shoulder blades.*

3. Heat activate the glue.

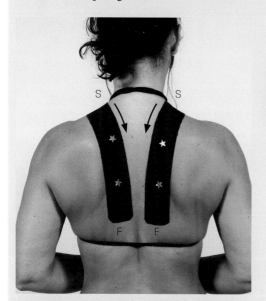

Figure 6.2 *First application of two "I" strips lengthwise between the shoulder blades.*

2. Apply two standard "I" strips across the mid-thoracic region between the shoulder blades and with 75% stretch to each strip (Fig. 6.3).

Thoracic back pain and rhomboids

POSTERIOR CERVICAL PAIN

The following technique is fantastic for helping to reduce pain to the area posterior to the neck. If a patient complains of pain to the base of the neck, and it is on both sides, then the following technique is perfect as it can really help reduce their symptoms. There are a multitude of causes for this type of pain. Many of my patients have muscle pain or a perceived muscular tightness, which is often due to habitual movements/lifestyle and is a routine source of discomfort (Fig. 6.4).

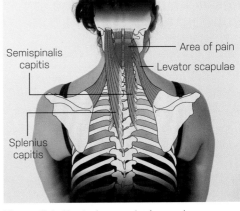

Figure 6.4 *Posterior cervical muscles.*

1. Place the cervical spine into flexion so that the posterior cervical muscles are on stretch. Apply two standard "I" strips starting from the base of the hairline and continue down along the erector spinae muscle, with 25% stretch to each strip (Fig. 6.5).

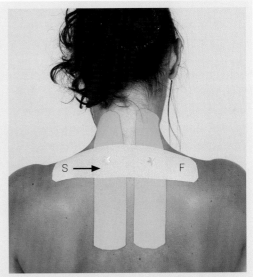

Figure 6.6 *Second application of one "I" strip across the area of pain.*

3. Heat activate the glue.

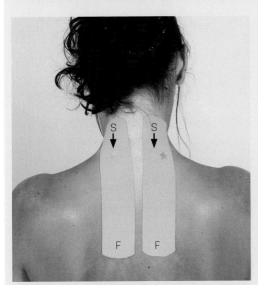

Figure 6.5 *First application of two "I" strips to the posterior part of the neck.*

2. Apply one standard "I" strip across the area of pain with 75% stretch (Fig. 6.6).

Neck and upper back pain

CERVICAL SPINE: LEVATOR SCAPULAE/UPPER TRAPEZIUS STRAIN

González-Iglesias et al. (2009) conducted the study "Short-term effects of cervical Kinesio Taping on pain and cervical ROM in patients with acute whiplash injury." They concluded that when patients presented with acute whiplash-associated conditions, kinesiology taping exhibited statistically significant improvements immediately following application and at a 24-hour follow-up.

At the superior angle of the scapula is the attachment of the levator scapulae muscle; therefore, one might presume when a patient presents with pain to this area that the muscle is the problem. I agree that this muscle might be part of the whole picture of the patient's symptoms, but one must also consider what other structures may be involved. For example, the facet joints of the cervical spine; other muscles like the trapezius, the rhomboids, or even the supraspinatus; and a first rib dysfunction should be considered (Fig. 6.7).

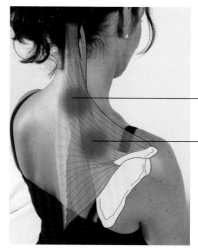

Trapezius strain

Levator scapulae strain

Figure 6.7 *Pain located to the superior angle of the scapulae and a strain of the upper trapezius muscle.*

1. Place the levator scapulae on stretch by side bending and rotating the neck to the opposite side from the pain. Apply one "Y" strip from the inferior aspect of scapula toward the origin of the levator scapulae, with little to no stretch of the tape (Fig. 6.8).
2. Ask the patient to slightly retract their shoulder. Apply the second "Y" strip starting from the supraclavicular fossa and tension the tape across the trapezius one leg at a time, at 75% stretch (Fig. 6.9).

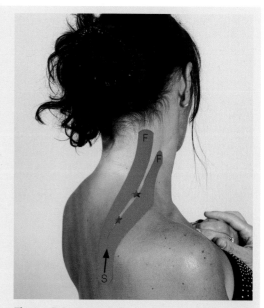

Figure 6.8 *First application to the levator scapulae muscle.*

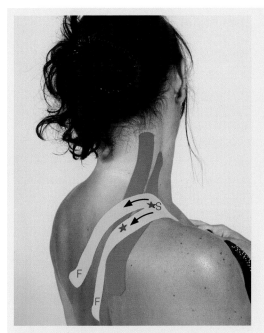

Figure 6.9 *Second application to the trapezius muscle.*

3. Heat activate the glue.

Neck/trapezius and levator scapulae pain

POSTURAL TAPING

One of the questions patients and athletes regularly ask me is "What do you think of my posture?" or "Is my posture bad?"

The following are three techniques I would personally recommend, as they have been very effective when implemented at my clinic in Oxford.

Technique 1

This technique is probably the easiest option and potentially the most effective, as I have found that *the simple approach is sometimes the best approach.*

1. The patient is sitting and they are asked to retract their shoulders slightly to activate their rhomboids. The therapist splits the tape in the middle and peels some of the tape back and then applies the Big Daddy tape to the center of the patient's back. The therapist locks the center of the tape and then increases the tension to 75% and lays it down across the scapula, as shown in Figure 6.10.

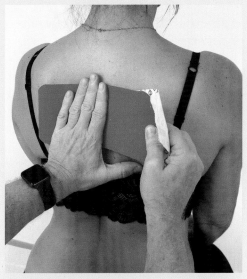

Figure 6.10 *Therapist applies the Big Daddy tape across one scapula.*

2. Next, the therapist locks the center of the tape and then increases the tension to 75% and lays it down across the other scapula, as shown in Figure 6.11 (a&b).

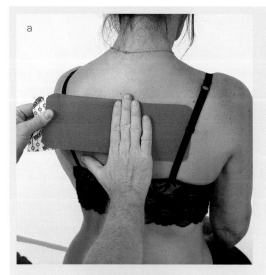

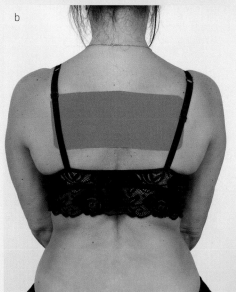

Figure 6.11 a: *Therapist applies the Big Daddy tape across the other scapula with 75% tension.* **b:** *Finished technique.*

3. Heat activate the glue.

Technique 2

The following technique is a continuation of the above. You have a choice: apply the following tape in conjunction with the Big Daddy (above) or, if you prefer, you can use the two postural strips without the larger central tape. I decide by what my patients say to me; if they feel they need more stability then I will use both techniques.

1. The therapist cuts two longer "I" strips and applies the first one from the supraclavicular fossa (above the clavicle). The patient is asked to pull their shoulders back and down to promote a better posture. The therapist then increases the tension to 75% and lays the tape down toward their lower back, as shown in Figure 6.12.

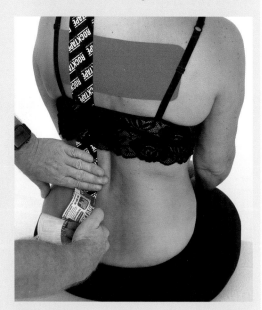

Figure 6.12 *Therapist applies the postural strip toward the lumbar spine with 75% tension.*

2. Next, the therapist applies the tape to the opposite supraclavicular fossa and repeats the same process, as shown in Figure 6.13 (a&b).

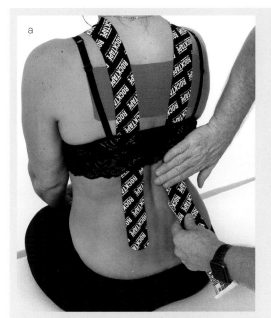

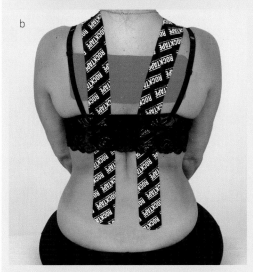

Figure 6.13 a: *Therapist applies the postural strip toward the lumbar spine with 75% tension.* **b:** *Finished technique.*

3. Heat activate the glue.

Thoracic back pain (using Big Daddy)

Technique 3

The following technique is an alternative to the above. Some patients prefer this method because some of the postural braces you can purchase have a *crossing* effect.

1. The therapist cuts two longer "I" strips and applies the first one from the supraclavicular fossa (above the clavicle). The patient is asked to pull their shoulders back and down to promote a better posture. The therapist increases the tension to 75% and lays it down across the middle part of their back and toward the opposite lumbar spine. The same is repeated on the other side, as shown in Figure 6.14.

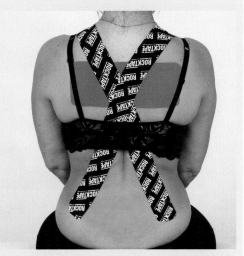

Figure 6.14 *Therapist applies the postural strips toward the opposite lumbar spine with 75% tension.*

2. Heat activate the glue.

Postural taping— cross technique

PECTORAL STRAIN

Tape is seldom applied to the pectoral muscles because this area of the body is particularly awkward to apply tape to, especially with females, and because therapists do not often actually treat strains to these muscles. On occasion during my courses I have been asked if I can teach the taping technique to the pectorals, or for a rare condition to the rib called costochondritis. In the latter condition it is possible that taping might help reduce some of the pain.

1. The patient is supine and is asked to place their arm to the side so that the pectorals are on stretch and then to place their other hand on the top of their chest (females). The therapist applies the first "I" strip to the sternal fibers of the pectoralis major and lays down the tape with little to no stretch to the insertion point on the humerus, as shown in Figure 6.15.

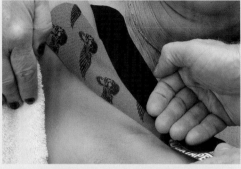

Figure 6.16a *Therapist applies the first strip with no stretch from the clavicular fibers to the insertion point.*

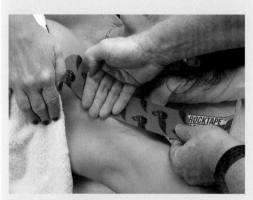

Figure 6.15 *Therapist applies the first strip with no stretch from the sternal fibers to the insertion point.*

2. The therapist applies the second "I" strip to the clavicular fibers of the pectoralis major and lays down the tape with little to no stretch to the insertion point on the humerus, as shown in Figure 6.16 (a&b).

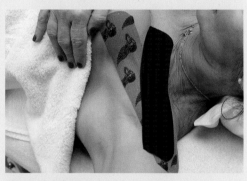

Figure 6.16b *Finished technique.*

3. Heat activate the glue.

Pectoral muscle taping

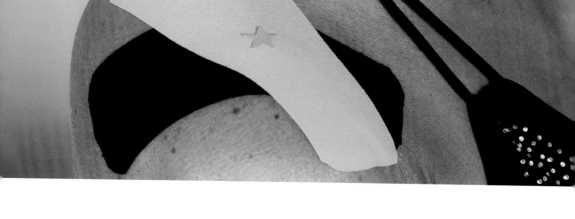

CHAPTER 7

KINESIOLOGY TAPING TECHNIQUES FOR THE UPPER LIMBS

ROTATOR CUFF TENDINOPATHY: SUPRASPINATUS, BURSITIS, AND INFRASPINATUS PAIN

Kaya et al. (2010) compared Kinesio Taping to physical therapy modalities for the treatment of shoulder impingement syndrome. They concluded that Kinesio Taping could be an alternative treatment option for shoulder impingement syndrome, especially when an immediate effect is needed.

In addition, Hsu et al. (2009) investigated the effect of Kinesio Taping on shoulder impingement syndrome in baseball players. They found that the activation of the lower fibers of the trapezius, when returning the arm from a scapulohumeral rhythm, increased during the 60–30° lowering phase of the arm.

So where do I start in terms of the shoulder? (For more in-depth information, please read my book, *The Vital Shoulder Complex: An Illustrated Guide to Assessment, Treatment, and Rehabilitation*.) Currently, my preference is for the following taping technique as the tape can be modified depending on the soft tissue that is presenting the pain. As an example, if the patient has localized pain to the anterior aspect of the shoulder then it could be a supraspinatus tendinopathy that is the problem. Pain inferior to the acromion could well be a subacromial bursa, and pain posterior to the greater tubercle of the humerus might indicate an issue with the infraspinatus muscle, especially if this patient is a swimmer.

Figure 7.1 shows the three potential areas of pain that relate to the shoulder, as mentioned above.

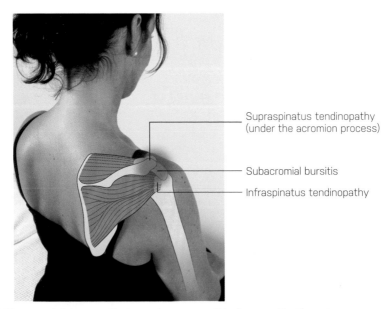

Supraspinatus tendinopathy
(under the acromion process)

Subacromial bursitis

Infraspinatus tendinopathy

Figure 7.1 *Three painful areas that can be responsible for a patient's pain.*

1. The first technique is applied to help offload the deltoid muscle. If any shoulder issues are present then this technique is generally done first. Apply a "Y" strip from the deltoid tuberosity, place the anterior deltoid into a stretched position and apply one tail of the tape to the anterior deltoid. Then place the posterior deltoid into a stretch and apply the second tail of the tape to the posterior deltoid, with little to no stretch (Fig. 7.2).

2. Ask the patient to place their hand onto their lower back, as this will stretch the supraspinatus and the infraspinatus muscles. Apply a "Y" strip from the area of pain: start at the anterior aspect of the shoulder to cover the supraspinatus, the inferior aspect of the acromion for the bursa, and the posterior aspect of the greater tubercle of the humerus for the infraspinatus (Fig. 7.3). Each tail of the tape

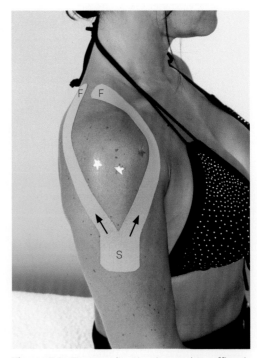

Figure 7.2 *First application is used to offload the deltoid muscle.*

is applied with a 75% stretch. You can also ask the patient to retract their shoulder slightly as this will enhance its position prior to the application of the tape.

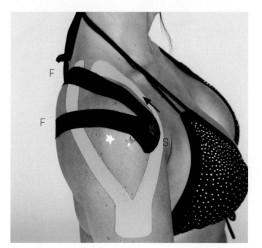

Figure 7.3 *Second application to cover the specific area of pain.*

3. Heat activate the glue.

Shoulder pain/rotator cuff and bursitis

ACROMIOCLAVICULAR JOINT SPRAIN

When I was a physical therapist working with a rugby team, sprains of the acromioclavicular joint (ACJ) were a regular occurrence, almost to the point that I would see some type of injury to this joint at almost every training session and game. As rugby is a contact game, subluxations/sprains from this sport are regularly seen by physical therapists (Fig. 7.4). ACJ sprains are not exclusive to rugby, as most sports can, at some point, involve this joint: I subluxed my left ACJ many years ago while kayaking on a particularly fast river in Germany. This area is tricky to treat as the patient finds it difficult to rest the shoulder because even getting dressed requires movement

from this part of the body, not to mention the fact that athletes like to keep active. Hence, the following kinesiology taping technique is a perfect option as it assists the healing mechanism.

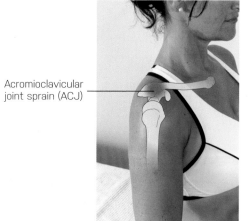

Acromioclavicular joint sprain (ACJ)

Figure 7.4 *ACJ sprain.*

1. Place the patient's arm by their side so that there is no stretch applied to the ACJ. Apply a standard "I" strip across the ACJ with 75–100% stretch of the tape (Fig. 7.5).

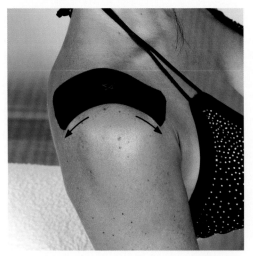

Figure 7.5 *First application of an "I" strip across the ACJ.*

2. Apply another standard "I" strip with 75–100% stretch (Fig. 7.6).

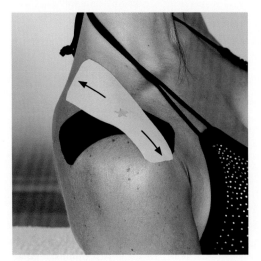

Figure 7.6 *Second application of an "I" strip across the ACJ.*

3. Apply a third standard "I" strip with 75–100% stretch (Fig. 7.7).

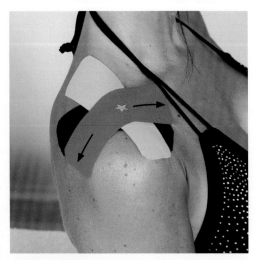

Figure 7.7 *Third application of an "I" strip across the ACJ.*

4. Heat activate the glue.

Shoulder pain/ACJ

BICEPS: LONG HEAD AND SHORT HEAD

Fratocchi et al. (2012) conducted a study to see if Kinesio Taping applied over the biceps brachii influenced isokinetic elbow peak torque. They concluded that there was indeed an increase in the concentric elbow peak torque for a group of healthy subjects.

Pain at the anterior aspect of the shoulder, as mentioned earlier, could be coming from the supraspinatus tendon. However, it could also be a tendinopathy of the long head of the biceps as this structure originates from the supraglenoid tubercle, penetrates through the shoulder structures, continues through the bicipital groove, and finally attaches to the radius and the bicipital aponeurosis (Fig. 7.8). Ruptures of the long head are relatively common in men over 45 years. This is known as a "Popeye" arm as the rupture causes recoil and subsequently gives the appearance of an increased lump when the biceps is contracted.

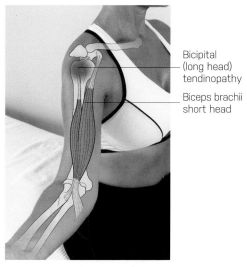

Bicipital (long head) tendinopathy

Biceps brachii short head

Figure 7.8 *Bicipital tendinopathy of the long head of the biceps.*

1. Place the biceps muscle into a stretched position and apply a "Y" strip, with little to no stretch, starting from the insertion point on the radius. The tails of the tape are applied to the long head and the short head of the biceps respectively (Fig. 7.9).
2. Apply a smaller than standard "I" strip with 75–100% stretch across the area of pain (Fig. 7.10).

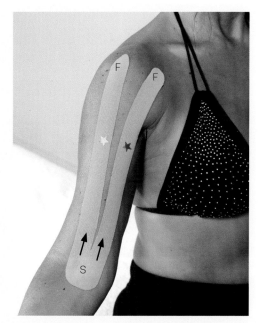

Figure 7.9 *First application of a "Y" strip covering both heads of the biceps.*

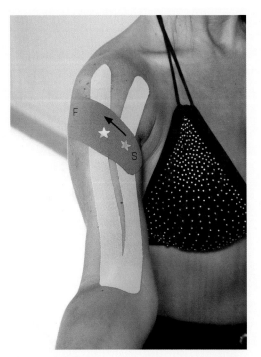

Figure 7.10 *Second application of a small "I" strip across the area of pain.*

3. Heat activate the glue.

Shoulder and biceps pain

CHAPTER 8

KINESIOLOGY TAPING TECHNIQUES FOR THE FOREARM, HAND, AND WRIST

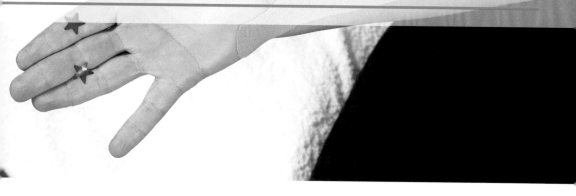

LATERAL EPICONDYLITIS: TENNIS ELBOW

Elbow pain, especially on the lateral side, can be very intense and debilitating for patients. Sometimes even just lifting a coffee cup can cause excruciating pain. When applying kinesiology tape to this area of pain, ensure that it is not a referred pattern of pain coming from the cervical spine (C6/C7) rather than directly from the elbow.

One simple test I ask my patients to do, to confirm that it is a muscular issue and not a referred pain, is to resist extension of the middle finger. If this particular test is painful at the lateral part of the elbow, then it will usually confirm that the tendon responsible for the pain is the extensor carpi radialis brevis (ECRB).

This muscle has an origin at the lateral epicondyle (common extensor origin) and inserts onto the middle metacarpal bone; hence, the reasoning behind extension of the middle finger. Figure 8.1 shows the ECRB.

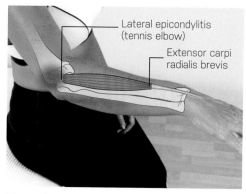

Figure 8.1 *Most common muscle responsible for tennis elbow.*

1. Using a longer "I" strip, fold one square of the tape over another and cut out two small "kite" shapes (Fig. 8.2).

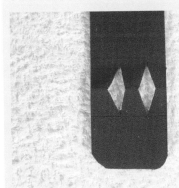

Figure 8.2 *Two "kite"-shaped cutouts.*

2. Insert the index and middle finger of the patient's hand through the two cutouts. Then place the elbow into pronation and extension with the wrist placed into flexion. Apply the tape along the length of the ECRB tendon to the attachment on the lateral epicondyle, with little to no stretch (Fig. 8.3).

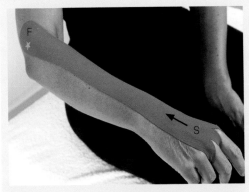

Figure 8.3 *First application using a longer "I" strip.*

3. Using a "Y" strip, attach the kinesiology tape slightly posterior to the lateral epicondyle and apply 75–100% stretch to each of the tails so that they cross the initial "I" strip. Each of the "tails" should finish on the flexor side of the forearm (Fig. 8.4).

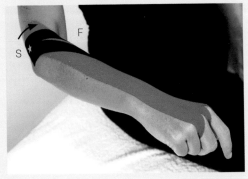

Figure 8.4 *Second application of a "Y" strip.*

4. Heat activate the glue.

Tennis elbow

MEDIAL EPICONDYLITIS AND ULNAR NERVE: GOLFER'S ELBOW

When I was a physical trainer with the army I liked climbing ropes as I found this exercise very effective for building my strength. However, over time I would feel pain to the inside aspect of my elbow and I was told I had golfer's elbow, even though I did not play golf. This condition can basically affect anybody, and it is normally caused by one particular muscle, pronator teres (Fig. 8.5). This muscle originates at the medial epicondyle; hence, the term "medial epicondylitis." There is also a relationship to the ulnar nerve due to the proximity of the inflammation. If a patient perceives a tingling or altered sensation to their little finger then the ulnar nerve is also involved.

The following kinesiology taping technique will help both the pronator teres and the ulnar nerve.

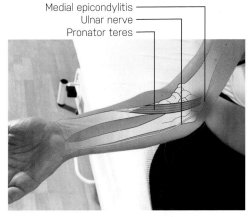

Figure 8.5 *Pronator teres and its relationship to the ulnar nerve.*

1. Place the pronator teres muscle into a stretched position by supinating the forearm and extending the elbow. Then apply an "I" strip, with little to no stretch, starting from the origin point on the medial epicondyle and finishing across the pronator teres (Fig. 8.6).

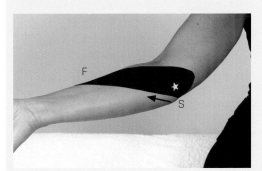

Figure 8.6 *First application of an "I" strip to the pronator teres.*

2. Apply a smaller than standard "Y" strip, with 75–100% stretch, across the area of pain (Fig. 8.7).

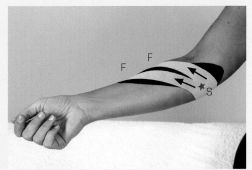

Figure 8.7 *Second application of a smaller "Y" strip across the area of pain.*

3. Heat activate the glue.

Golfer's elbow/ ulnar nerve

CARPAL TUNNEL SYNDROME

The carpal tunnel is located between the four palpable bones in the wrist, called the pisiform, hamate, scaphoid, and trapezium. Through this tunnel pass the median nerve and the superficial and deep flexor finger tendons. Carpal tunnel syndrome is basically a compression of the median nerve, and one particular cause of this syndrome is an overuse condition called "tenosynovitis" of the flexor tendons. The tendons become inflamed and subsequently cause a compression of the nerve with altered sensations to the thumb, index and middle fingers, as well as half of the ring finger (Fig. 8.8). Kinesiology taping can help reduce both the swelling of the flexors and the pain in the hand and fingers.

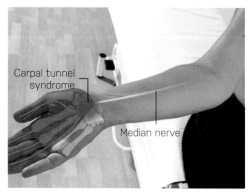

Figure 8.8 *Carpal tunnel syndrome.*

1. Ask the patient to gently stretch their flexor tendons by extending their wrist and elbow. Apply a modified "I" strip with a small tail cut at either end so that it looks like a long "X" shape. This should be applied with little to no stretch (Fig. 8.9).

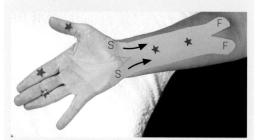

Figure 8.9 *Application of the tape to reduce the symptoms of carpal tunnel syndrome.*

2. Heat activate the glue.

Carpal tunnel syndrome

INTERSECTION SYNDROME AND DE QUERVAIN'S TENDINOSIS

There are two specific conditions in particular that I feel kinesiology taping can help. One injury is very common with rowers and is called intersection syndrome: typically developed by the "feathering hand" as a result of the sweep stroke in rowing. The second condition affects the extensor pollicis brevis and abductor pollicis longus and is called De Quervain's tendinosis. Figure 8.10 shows these two conditions of the wrist.

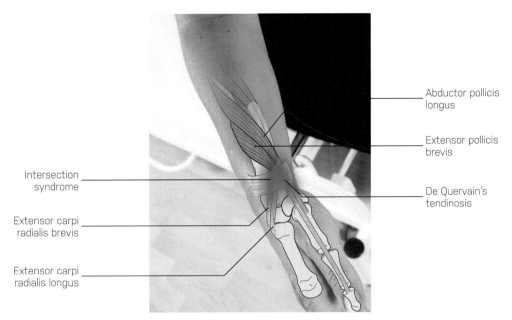

Figure 8.10 *De Quervain's tendinosis and intersection syndrome.*

1. Ask the patient to gently place their wrist into ulnar deviation as this will place the thumb tendons on stretch. Apply a small "I" strip starting from the first metacarpophalangeal (MCP) joint and continue toward the thumb tendons and the area of pain, with little to no stretch (Fig. 8.11).

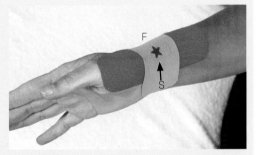

Figure 8.12 *Second application across the area of pain to provide decompression.*

3. Heat activate the glue.

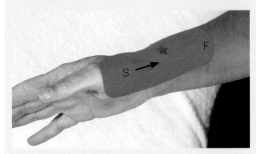

Tendinitis of wrist and forearm

Figure 8.11 *First application of an "I" strip along the thumb tendons.*

2. Apply another small "I" strip across the area of pain with 75–100% stretch of the tape (Fig. 8.12).

OSTEOARTHRITIS (OA) OF THE FIRST CARPOMETACARPAL (CMC) JOINT

Perhaps surprisingly, it is the base of the thumb that is considered to be the first joint in the body that will suffer with arthritis, and potentially 30–40% of all men and women between the ages of 50 and 60 years old will suffer with this condition. I often ask massage therapists to be careful during treatments as too much use of the thumb might lead to early degenerative changes.

The pain is located at the base of the thumb. This is known as the saddle joint, and it lies between the trapezium (carpal bone) and the first metacarpal, as shown in Figure 8.13.

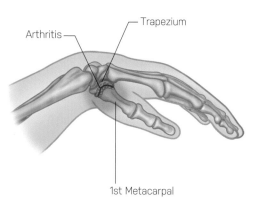

Figure 8.13 *Osteoarthritis of the first carpometacarpal joint.*

To apply kinesiology tape to this area we will need the following: 3 × "I" strips, one of which will have a small "kite" shape cut out, as shown in Figure 8.14.

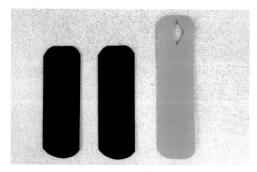

Figure 8.14 *Three small "I" strips, one cut with a kite shape.*

1. Ask the patient to gently open their fingers and to place the thumb into slight flexion. Apply the small "I" strip with the kite shape directly over the thumb and gently tension to tape and finish across the CMC joint and continue toward the thumb tendons, as shown in Figure 8.15.

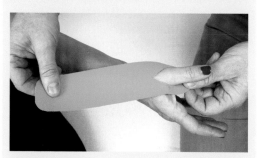

Figure 8.15 *First application of an "I" strip (with the kite) along the base of the thumb.*

2. Next, apply another small "I" strip: start from the dorsal hand and finish across the base of the thumb with 50–75% stretch of the tape (Fig. 8.16).

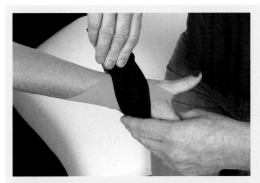

Figure 8.16 *Apply another small "I" strip.*

3. Apply another small "I" strip: start from the thenar eminence of the thumb and continue and finish across the base of the thumb with 50–75% stretch of the tape (Fig. 8.17).

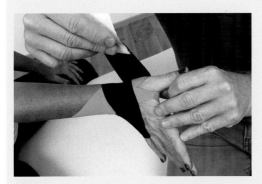

Figure 8.17 *Apply another small "I" strip.*

4. Heat activate the glue.

Once you have applied the three "I" small strips then the finished result should look like Figure 8.18.

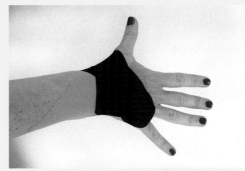

Figure 8.18 *Three taping applications applied to the base of the thumb.*

Arthritic thumb (OA)

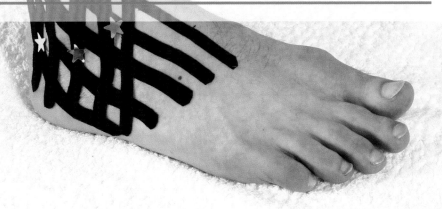

CHAPTER 9

KINESIOLOGY TAPING TECHNIQUES TO CONTROL EDEMA (SWELLING)

LYMPHATIC SYSTEM

The lymphatic system is a unique, one-way system and is commonly called the body's "drainage" mechanism. It is a subset of the circulatory system and comprises a network of organs, lymphatic vessels, and small structures known as lymph nodes (Fig. 9.1). The lymphatic system carries a clear, colorless fluid called "lymph" back toward the heart. This system has many functions, including the removal of excessive interstitial fluid: this is the extracellular fluid that accumulates within most of the body's tissues and is returned as lymph fluid, via vessels, back to the cardiovascular system.

On the route back toward the circulatory system the lymph fluid is forced through the lymph nodes so that it can be filtered. Within these nodes there are specialized white blood cells, called "lymphocytes," and their purpose is to destroy any harmful organisms that have been trapped within the nodes. Lymphocyte cells are also added to the lymph fluid that flows out of the nodes and back to the bloodstream. Another function of the lymphatic system is to absorb and transport lipids from the digestive system to the venous circulation.

The following kinesiology taping techniques are an excellent way of helping to reduce any form of swelling/edema that has accumulated within the soft tissues. A physical therapist colleague of mine treated a lady who had undergone a

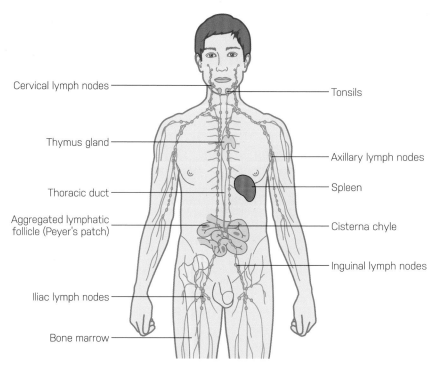

Figure 9.1 *Diagram of the lymphatic system.*

mastectomy (breast removal); she also had some of her axillary lymph nodes removed as a precaution. This patient suffered with occasional swelling to her arm as a result of the lymph nodes being removed. My colleague applied this specific type of kinesiology taping to her swollen arm and within a short period the swelling had reduced and so had the pain.

Tsai et al. (2009) conducted a study and asked the question "Could kinesio tape replace the bandage in decongestive lymphatic therapy for breast cancer related lymphedema?" The study results showed that kinesio tape could be a replacement and they also found that the acceptance of this tape was better than

for the bandage due to longer wearing time, less difficulty in usage, and increased comfort and convenience. The results also demonstrated a significant reduction in swelling/edema (i.e., excess water) with the use of kinesio tape. In addition, Bialoszewski et al. (2009) investigated the clinical efficacy of kinesiology taping for reducing edema in the lower limbs. The results showed that the application of kinesiology tape produced a statistically significant decrease in the circumference of the thigh when compared to the standard treatment group.

The following kinesiology taping techniques are all very similar in appearance. Once the basic principles and applications have been learnt, this type of technique can be applied to anywhere on the body that would benefit the patient, especially if there is some form of swelling of the underlying tissues.

One of my patients is a rowing coach at Oxford University. She has had a full replacement of her right knee and, due to her continually active job coaching the rowing team, she has regular swelling to this area. After a long treatment session, she informed me that out of all the physical therapy techniques I use to treat her—e.g., osteopathy, sports therapy and acupuncture—when I apply the kinesiology taping technique this has the best results in terms of reducing her pain and swelling. Why? The main difference is that the kinesiology tape is left on for up to five days, so the tape is working "24/7," and is especially effective while she is sleeping.

I have been known to say to my students, during kinesiology taping lectures, that once these techniques are learnt they will completely change their lives for the better, especially in terms of treating their athletes and patients. I have also mentioned time and time again during classes that I spent 5 years of my life, and a serious amount of money, becoming an osteopath, and yet I have had better effects with my patients and athletes at times when I have only applied the kinesiology tape. This usually amuses my students, but once they have started to use these techniques with patients they often agree with my comments.

The following taping techniques, as previously mentioned, have a similar appearance once the tape has been applied to the body part. The kinesiology tape is normally cut into an "I" strip, then the tape is cut into five equal tails, or what I call "fingers" (Fig. 9.2), although the tape can also be cut into four fingers if preferred. I personally find that five fingers have better effects, but it is up to personal preference. The piece of tape is now referred to as a "fan." Using scissors, round off the end of each finger so that it does not lift away when clothes are taken on/off, etc. The "pad" (beginning) of the tape, before it eventually becomes the individual fingers, is placed toward the area of the relevant lymphatic nodes.

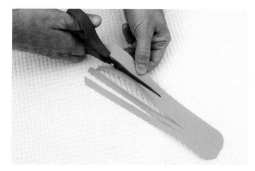

Figure 9.2 *An "I" strip being cut into the shape of a "fan."*

The kinesiology tape can be applied to the area of the body with no stretch of the body's tissue and no stretch of the tape, it is simply laid down over the area of swelling with little to no stretch. However, I do place the ankle and knee into a slightly stretched position before I apply the tape, but only to the point where there is no discomfort to the patient. Remember my saying from earlier: "Swelling causes pressure and pressure causes pain."

ANKLE EDEMA

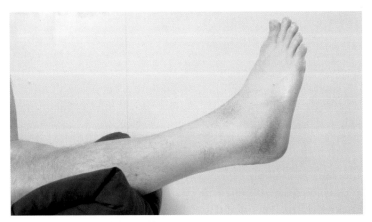

Figure 9.3 *A common swelling of the ankle joint.*

1. Ask the patient to place their ankle into a slight stretch by encouraging the motion called inversion, but only a small movement is needed. If this motion is too painful for your patient then simply apply the kinesiology tape to the ankle with no stretch applied to the ankle joint.
2. Start the first application of the tape superior and lateral to the lateral malleolus (distal fibula). Apply the pad with no stretch and place the individual fingers across the area of swelling (Fig. 9.4).

3. Apply the second kinesiology "fan" tape superiorly and medially to the lateral malleolus. Then place each finger across the tape from the first application, with little to no stretch (Fig. 9.5). The shape of a "lattice" should be seen.

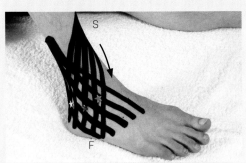

Figure 9.5 *Second application of the kinesiology tape is placed across the first piece of tape.*

4. Heat activate the glue and be careful not to lift each of the fingers.

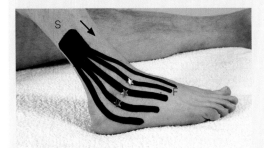

Figure 9.4 *First application, the individual fingers are laid across the area of swelling with no stretch.*

Ankle edema

KNEE EDEMA

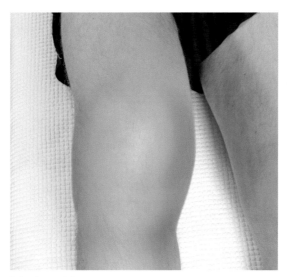

Figure 9.6 *Swelling of the knee joint.*

1. Place the knee into flexion and apply the first fan shape from the medial side of the lower thigh. Lay the fingers across the knee with little to no stretch (Fig. 9.7).

2. Repeat the same technique, but this time start from the lateral side of the lower thigh. Lay down the fingers across the first application (Fig. 9.8)

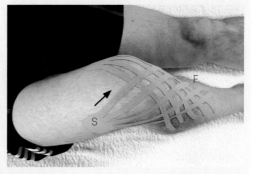

Figure 9.8 *Second application of the "fan" tape is placed across the first technique.*

3. Heat activate the glue.

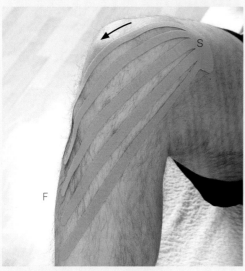

Figure 9.7 *First application of the "fan" across the knee.*

Swollen (edema) knee

HEMATOMA/EDEMA OF THE THIGH

What you might consider to be a simple bruise or what an athlete may describe as a "dead leg" can actually be an "intramuscular hematoma" (i.e., bleeding within the muscle compartment) edema (Fig. 9.9). If left untreated, or indeed if treatment is over enthusiastic, this could lead to a more complicated condition called a "myositis ossificans." This condition, as the name suggests, causes the soft tissues (i.e., muscles) to potentially ossify (become bone), and it is a condition that should be strongly avoided. The next time a patient presents with a "dead leg," be cautious as it could be something a lot more serious.

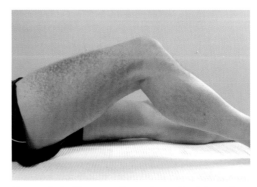

Figure 9.9 *Shows a hematoma/bruising of the anterior/lateral thigh.*

1. Place the knee into slight flexion as this puts the quadriceps onto a gentle stretch. Apply the first fan shape from the lateral side of the upper thigh and place the fingers across toward the medial lower side of the thigh, with little to no stretch (Fig. 9.10).

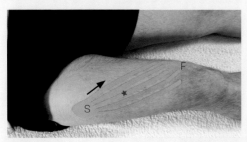

Figure 9.10 *First application of the "fan" across the hematoma.*

2. Repeat the same technique, but this time start from the medial side of the upper thigh. Lay down the fingers across the first application (Fig. 9.11).

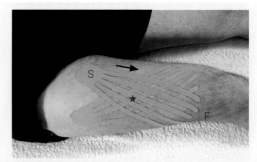

Figure 9.11 *Second application of the "fan" tape is placed across the first technique.*

3. Heat activate the glue.

Thigh edema

FOREARM EDEMA

I was first shown this technique by a student who was on my kinesiology course in Ireland. She was a professional motorcyclist and demonstrated a technique used by a physiotherapist, before every event, as a preventative measure for a condition called "muscular pump" of the forearms. I have now used this technique numerous times with the rowers at Oxford, as it also helps reduce the possibility of pain caused by "compartment syndrome" (Fig. 9.12) within the flexors of the forearms.

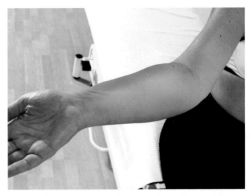

Figure 9.12 *Swelling/compartment syndrome of the flexors.*

1. Place the wrist and elbow into extension and apply the first fan shape from the lateral side of the forearm. Lay the fingers across the forearm flexors, with little to no stretch (Fig. 9.13).

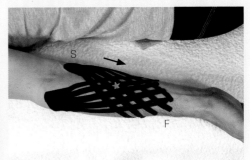

Figure 9.14 *Second application of the "fan" tape is placed across the first application.*

3. Heat activate the glue.

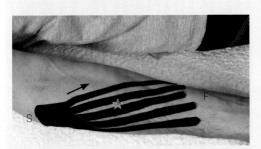

Figure 9.13 *First application of the "fan" across the flexors of the forearm.*

2. Repeat the same technique, but this time start from the posterior side of the shoulder joint and lay down the fingers across the first application (Fig. 9.14).

Flexor compartment/ muscle pump syndrome

SHOULDER EDEMA

Swelling of the shoulder is quite rare to see by comparison to the ankle joint, where swelling is a bit more obvious. If a patient has pain all over the shoulder joint, i.e., not localized to one area, then this next technique will work very well to help reduce the swelling and pain (Fig. 9.15). Patients who have "capsulitis," more commonly known as a "frozen shoulder," will have pain affecting the whole of the shoulder due to the involvement of the capsule, so this technique, in my experience, can really be helpful.

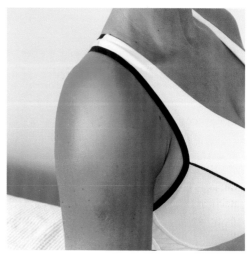

Figure 9.15 *General swelling of the shoulder joint.*

1. Place the patient's arm by the side of their body with no stretch to the shoulder muscles. Apply the first fan shape from the anterior aspect of the shoulder near the coracoid process. Lay the fingers across the area of pain across the shoulder joint, with little to no stretch (Fig. 9.16).

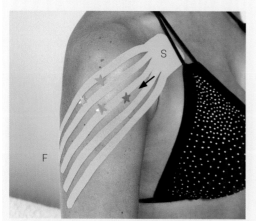

Figure 9.16 *First application of the "fan" across the anterior shoulder joint.*

2. Repeat the same technique, but this time start from the posterior side of the

shoulder joint and lay down the fingers across the first application (Fig. 9.17).

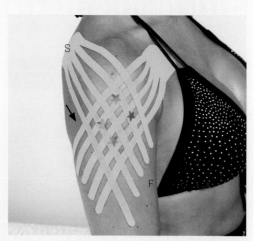

Figure 9.17 *Second application of the "fan" tape is placed across the first application.*

3. Heat activate the glue.

Shoulder/rotator cuff edema

BIBLIOGRAPHY

Aminaka N, Gribble PA 2008. Patellar taping, patellofemoral pain syndrome, lower extremity kinematics, and dynamic postural control. *Journal of Athletic Training* 43(1):21–28.

Bialoszewski D, Wozniak W, Zarek S 2009. Clinical efficacy of kinesiology taping in reducing edema of the lower limbs in patients treated with the Ilizarov method. *Orthopaedic Traumatology Rehabilitation* 11(1):46–54.

Bicici S, Karatas N, Baltaci G 2012. Effect of athletic taping and Kinesio Taping on measurements of functional performance in basketball players with chronic inversion ankle sprains. *The International Journal of Sports Physical Therapy* 7(2):154–66.

Capobianco S, van den Dries G 2009. *Power Taping, 2nd edn*, Rocktape inc., USA.

Castro-Sanchez AM, Lara-Paloma IC, Mataran-Penarrocha GA et al. 2012. Kinesio Taping reduces disability and pain slightly in chronic non-specific low back pain: a randomised trial. *Journal of Physiotherapy* 58(2):89–95.

Chen PL, Hong WH, Lin CH et al. 2008. Biomechanics effects of Kinesio Taping for persons with patellofemoral pain syndrome during stair climbing. *Biomedical* 21:395–97.

Earls J, Myers T 2017. *Fascial Release for Structural Balance*. Lotus Publishing, Chichester, UK.

Fratocchi G, Mattia FD, Rossi R et al. 2012. Influence of Kinesio Taping applied over biceps brachii on isokinetic elbow peak torque. A placebo controlled study in a population of young healthy subjects. *Journal of Science and Medicine in Sport* 16(3):245–49.

Gibbons J 2022. *Muscle Energy Techniques: A Practical Guide for Physical Therapists.* Lotus Publishing, Chichester, UK.

Gonzalez-Iglesias J, Fernandez-de-les-Penas C, Cleland J et al. 2009. Short term effects of cervical kinesiology taping on pain and cervical range of motion in patients with acute whiplash injury: a randomized clinical trial. *Journal of Orthopaedic and Sports Physical Therapy* 39(7):515–21.

Hsu YH, Chen WY, Lin HC et al. 2009. The effects of taping on scapula kinematics and muscle performance in baseball players with shoulder impingement syndrome. *Journal of Electromyography and Kinesiology* 19(6):1092–99.

Huijing P 2009. Epimuscular myofascial force transmission: a historical perspective and implications for new research. *Journal of Biomechanics* 42:9–21.

Huijing P, Baan G 2008. Myofascial force trsnsmission via extramuscular pathways occurs between antagonistic muscles. *Cells Tissues Organs* 188:400–14.

Karatas N, Bicici S, Baltaci G et al. 2011. The effect of kinesio tape application on functional performance in surgeons who have musculo-skeletal pain after performing surgery. *Turkish Neurosurgery* 22(1):83–89.

Kase K, Tatsuyuki H, Tomoko O 1996. *Development of Kinesio Tape. Kinesio Taping Manual.* Kinesio Taping Association 6:117–18.

Kase K, Wallis J, Kase T 2003. *Clinical Therapeutic Applications of the Kinesio Taping Method, 2nd edn.* Ken Ikai Co. Ltd, Tokyo

Kaya E, Zinnuroglu M, Tugcu I 2010. Kinesio Taping compared to physical therapy modalities for the treatment of shoulder impingement. *Clinical Rheumatology* 30(2):201–7.

Kremler E, van de Port I, Backx F et al. 2011. A systematic review on the treatment of acute ankle sprain: brace versus other functional treatment types. *Sports Medicine* 41(3):185–97.

Lee JH, Yoo WG, Lee KS 2010. Effects of head–neck rotation and Kinesio Taping of the flexor muscles on dominant hand grip strength. *Journal of Physical Therapy Science* 22:285–89.

Lee JH, Yoo WG, Lee KS 2012. Treatment of chronic Achilles tendon pain by Kinesio Taping in an amateur badminton player. *Physical Therapy in Sport* 13:115–19.

Lee YY, Chang HY, Chang YC et al. 2012. The effect of applied direction to Kinesio Taping in ankle muscle strength and flexibility. *30th Annual Conference in Biomechanics in Sports*, Melbourne.

Merino R, Mayorga D, Fernandez E et al. 2010. Effect of Kinesio Taping on hip and lower trunk range of motion in triathletes. *Journal of Sport and Health Research* 2(2):109–18.

Morris D, Jones D, Ryan H 2013. The clinical effects of Kinesio® Tex taping: a systematic review. *Physiotherapy Theory and Practice* 29(4):259–70.

Murray H, Husk L 2001. Effect of Kinesio Taping on proprioception in the ankle. *Journal of Orthopaedics & Sports Physical Therapy* 31:A–37.

Myers TW 2020. *Anatomy Trains: Myofascial Meridians for Manual and Movement Therapists.* Churchill Livingstone/Elsevier, Edinburgh.

Rocktape: http://rocktape.net; http://rocktape.com; (last accessed November 2013).

Schleip R, Findley TW, Chaitow L et al. 2012. *Fascia: the Tensional Network of the Human Body.* Churchill Livingstone/Elsevier Edinburgh.

Sporttape: http://www.sporttape.co.uk; (last accessed November 2013).

Thelen MD, Dauber JA, Stoneman PD 2008. The clinical efficacy of Kinesio Tape for shoulder pain: a randomized, double-blinded, clinical trial. *Journal of Orthopaedic & Sports Physical Therapy* 38(7):389–95.

Tiger K Tape: http://www.tigertapes.com; (last accessed November 2013).

Tsai CT, Chang WD, Lee JP 2010. Effects of short-term treatment with kinesiotaping for plantar fasciitis. *Journal of Musculoskeletal Pain* 18:71–80.

Tsai HJ, Hung HC, Yang JL 2009. Could kinesio tape replace the bandage in decongestive lymphatic therapy for breast-cancer related lymphedema? *Support Care Cancer* 17(11):1353–60.

Vithoulka I, Beneja A, Malliou P et al. 2010. The effects of Kinesio Taping on quadriceps strength during isokinetic exercises in non athlete women. *Isokinetics and Exercise Science* 18:1–6.

Yoshida A, Kahanov L 2007. The effect of Kinesio Taping on lower trunk range of motions. *Research in Sports Medicine: An International Journal* 15(2):103–12.